THE PREVENT AND REVERSE HEART DISEASE COOKBOOK

· · · · ·

Over 125 Delicious, Life-Changing, Plant-Based Recipes

ANN CRILE ESSELSTYN and **JANE ESSELSTYN**

AVERY

a member of Penguin Group (USA)

New York

Published by the Penguin Group
Penguin Group (USA) LLC
375 Hudson Street
New York, New York 10014

USA • Canada • UK • Ireland • Australia
New Zealand • India • South Africa • China

penguin.com
A Penguin Random House Company

Most Avery books are available at special quantity discounts for bulk purchase for sales promotions, premiums, fund-raising,
and educational needs. Special books or book excerpts also can be created to fit specific needs.
For details, write Special.Markets@us.penguingroup.com.

Library of Congress Cataloging-in-Publication Data
Esselstyn, Ann Crile.
The prevent and reverse heart disease cookbook : more than 125 delicious, life-changing,
plant-based recipes / Ann Crile Esselstyn, Jane Esselstyn.
p.   cm.
Companion volume to: Prevent and reverse heart disease. New York : Avery, 2007.
ISBN 978-1-58333-558-1 (paperback)
1. Coronary heart disease—Diet therapy—Recipes.   2. Coronary heart disease—Prevention.   3. Vegetarian cooking.
4. Natural foods.   I. Esselstyn, Jane.   II. Esselstyn, Caldwell B., 1933– Prevent and reverse heart disease.   III. Title.
RC685.C6E75   2014
641.5'6311—dc23   2014015575

Printed in the United States of America
15

Book design by Gretchen Achilles

THE PREVENT AND REVERSE HEART DISEASE COOKBOOK

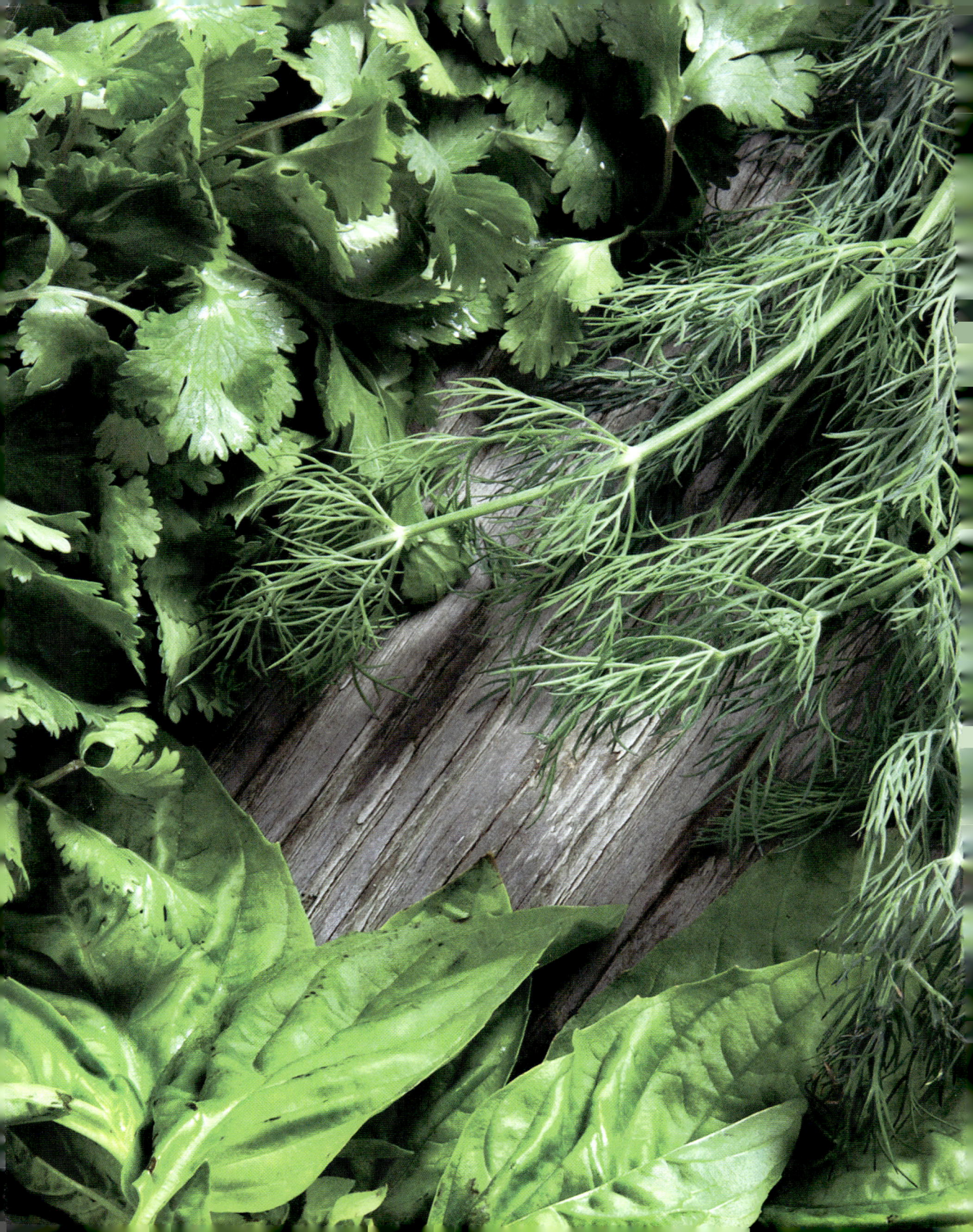

THIS BOOK IS DEDICATED TO
Bok choy,
Swiss chard,
kale,
collards,
collard greens,
beet greens,
mustard greens,
turnip greens,
Napa cabbage,
Brussels sprouts,
broccoli,
cauliflower,
cilantro,
parsley,
spinach,
arugula,
and asparagus.

But most especially to **Caldwell B. Esselstyn, Jr., MD,**
husband, father, and the voice behind it all.

And also to **Brian Hart**, husband, son-in law,
and the best cook in the family.

CONTENTS

THE PREVENT AND REVERSE HEART DISEASE COOKBOOK

FOREWORD

Just imagine that you and all of your loved ones could enjoy the treasured gift of lifelong health and wellness. This is not only possible, but it is at your fingertips this very moment through the recipes in *The Prevent and Reverse Heart Disease Cookbook*.

In 2007, I published *Prevent and Reverse Heart Disease*. I was driven to write this book because my research had shown that patients who had significant coronary artery heart disease could halt and reverse their illness simply by avoiding any oil, meat, and dairy products and eating whole food, plant-based nutrition.

My research, and the science behind whole food, plant-based nutrition, indicates that the endothelial cells, which line our blood vessels and are the life jacket and guardian of blood vessel health, are repeatedly injured from eating oils and animal-based foods.

I published the results of my original study in the *Journal of Family Practice* in 1995 and a twelve-year follow-up study in the *American Journal of Cardiology* in 1998. I wrote *Prevent and Reverse Heart Disease* in 2007 to share my groundbreaking findings more widely and to spread the message that by changing our nutrition, we can make ourselves heart-attack-proof.

It was gratifying when the book became a bestseller, reflecting the thirst for this breakthrough information. People rejoice when they become aware that *they* are empowered as the locus of control to halt and reverse a disease that has been destroying them.

There is broad evidence that plant-based nutrition is the key to abolishing chronic disease. Epidemiological studies of cultures that have traditionally plant-based diets confirm an absence of the common chronic diseases that kill so many Americans, such as heart disease, strokes, diabetes, hypertension, and obesity. These diseases and the drugs, procedures, and surgical interventions used for their treatment simply do not need to exist.

The strength of whole food, plant-based nutrition is further identified by studies of wartime deprivation. The 1951 study by Strom and Jansen [Mortality from circulatory diseases in Norway 1940–1945, *Lancet* (1951) 1: 126–129] highlighted the decrease in deaths from heart attacks and stroke in Norway during World War II, when the Axis powers of Germany confiscated Norwegian livestock and when Norwegians were, by necessity, consuming plant-based nutrition.

Naysayers state that patients will not follow or adhere to a major nutritional transition. On the contrary—our group's review of two hundred patients with significant cardiovascular disease, published in May 2014 by the *Journal of Family Practice*, found that nearly 90 percent of participants adhered to plant-based nutrition during the nearly four years of follow-up. We have found that the failure of other health professionals to achieve these results is not that the message is wrong but rather how the message is articulated.

There is nothing "radical" about a diet that most of the world follows by culture, heritage, and tradition, and that prevents the mortality, morbidity, and expense of treatment that accompanies common killing diseases. Economists estimate that eliminating heart disease would save the United States $40 trillion.

Recently, Cleveland Clinic cell biologist researchers discovered an additional way animal- and dairy-based foods injure arteries. Omnivores possess intestinal bacteria that convert ingested animal-based foods into trimethylamine N-oxide (TMAO). This molecule promotes vascular injury. People who consume plant-based foods simply do not possess the intestinal bacteria capable of making TMAO. These findings are yet another strong validation of the miraculous benefits of plant-based nutrition.

Just how transformative can plant-based nutrition be? Consider the story of Dick Dubois, a patient described in my first book. I first saw Dick in October 2005. A businessman and longtime triathlete, he was eventually crippled with angina (chest pain), which he experienced even during non-strenuous activities like merely walking to the mailbox. He was scheduled for heart bypass surgery but decided to try our plant-based nutrition plan in the months before his surgery.

Eleven days after Dick started eating according to our guidelines, his surgeon called to schedule the surgery for an earlier date. Dick declined. In just the eleven days he'd been following the plant-based nutrition plan, the chest pain he'd experienced while walking to the mailbox was completely gone!

His continued adherence to eating plant-based over eight and a half years has empowered his full recovery. Dick has been doing multiple triathlons yearly for the past five years. He even recently hiked in the Andes above 15,000 feet, all with his cardiologist's blessing. He never had the surgery. It was *just* the changes he made to his diet.

There are endless inspiring stories like these. People are experiencing how transformational—and delicious—plant-based nutrition is. They are giving up lifetime habits and refusing to eat food that is injuring them. And they are enjoying new tastes that also dramatically restore and maintain their health. Even if you don't suffer from heart disease, this nutritional lifestyle will give you optimal well-being. Three generations of our family are plant-based eaters and thriving. My wife, Ann, created all the wonderful recipes in my book *Prevent and Reverse Heart Disease*, and our daughter, Jane, did the same for all the delicious recipes in *My Beef with Meat*, by our son Rip. Now they're pooling their expertise and experience in this definitive cookbook.

My love and thanks to Ann and Jane for writing this quintessential cookbook, which has the power to change lives and help so many reclaim their health—a meritorious goal.

—Caldwell B. Esselstyn, Jr., MD

INTRODUCTION

We *love* our food! When all twenty of us Esselstyns gather together, our days are full of fun—biking, swimming, backflips off the dock, long runs, family baseball, and badminton. But we have the *most* fun cooking and eating together—the beautiful lasagnas, the rice-and-beans feasts, the nori-making sessions, the salads brimming with a rainbow of colors, the kale birthday cakes with blueberry frosting, and masses of curly, dinosaur, or Russian kale from the garden. Everyone cooks, even the grandchildren, whether they're ten or sixteen. The one person who doesn't cook is my husband. He is the permanent, full-time dishwasher.

When *Prevent and Reverse Heart Disease* was published in 2007 and went on to become a *New York Times* bestseller, it made an impact we couldn't even imagine. People all over the country and around the world heard the message that our family has lived by for years: Your health is truly in your own hands, and what you eat matters.

We've heard from people all over the United States and abroad whose lives have been changed by *Prevent and Reverse Heart Disease*. Why did it resonate? Because the program works, and because the science is irrefutable. In 1985, while a general surgeon at the Cleveland Clinic, my husband started a heart disease study with eighteen patients. Some of those patients were so sick they had been sent home to die. Incredibly, after twelve years, those patients were thriving on plant-based, no-oil diets. Twenty years later, compliant patients continued to thrive. Some still are thriving today in their late eighties. Eighty-eight-year-old Evelyn, one of those original patients, commented, "No one expected me to live! Here I am now, healthier than most of my friends." The wife of Anthony, another original patient, says, "Anthony thinks he will live forever, something none of us are privileged to do! He truly is steadfast in maintaining the plant-based diet and will not deviate under any circumstance."

We have worked with hundreds of patients since that original group, helping them take those first empowering steps toward reclaiming their health—all with the same miraculous results. My husband's research continues, and his most recent published study proves that when patients truly understand the power of nutrition, they are more than willing to change their diets. We have seen this firsthand—patients are always surprised how quickly they feel more energetic and healthy and how fast their cholesterol levels drop. And they can't believe how easy it is to put my husband's treatment guidelines into practice. They feel empowered being in control of reversing their disease.

The guidelines for those patients with heart disease are simple:

No meat
No dairy
No oil or nuts
Minimal salt and sweetener

What *can* you eat? A delicious and colorful array of vegetables, fruits, legumes, and whole grains, brimming with fiber, nutrients, and antioxidants, all great nourishment for your heart and your overall health.

In the last few years, spreading the word about the magic of plant-based nutrition has become a family affair. Our son Rip wrote the blockbuster bestsellers *The Engine 2 Diet* and *My Beef with Meat*, creating a national movement. And our daughter, Jane, created the recipe section for *My Beef with Meat*, which became a number-one *New York Times* bestseller. Rip calls his plan "plant-strong" and my husband's plan "plant-perfect." Both programs have no meat, dairy, or oil. Heart patients are also asked to eliminate nuts and avocado and to limit soy products.

A LIFE-CHANGING STORY

"My husband had his left circumflex artery stented in 2012. After talking to Dr. Esselstyn, my husband switched to the diet with full commitment and stopped having smoothies and flour and added a lot more greens than he had been eating, especially steamed kale.

"When he had the left circumflex artery stent, he also had a 100 percent blocked right coronary artery, which they did not stent that day. We were told that the blockage was severe and that the odds of success in opening the artery would be slim. They told us he'd have to go to a different facility for that second stent, six weeks later. Anticipating the procedure was horrible, but we were hopeful that, given the time on the diet between the two stents, some of the blockage might be reversed.

"I'd been told to expect a four- to five-hour surgery with two surgeons, but to my surprise, his surgery lasted only thirty minutes, with one surgeon! Only one catheter was needed, and no guide wires. The surgeon told us it was one of the easiest procedures he had ever done, and the head nurse said it was the quickest surgery of this type she'd ever seen.

"After six weeks on the diet, my husband's total cholesterol was 88, and his triglycerides were 110. I've been married to him for twenty-five years and never have his triglycerides been under 300. He and I truly believe that it was our focus on the diet that produced this happy outcome. My husband feels so much better today than he has in years. He's sworn to never again enter the hospital as a heart patient."

—DEBBIE H.

Jane is an excellent chef with a sophisticated palate. If I were left on my own, balsamic vinegar, mint, and cilantro would be in everything, and if something didn't taste right, I would go for the nutritional yeast. Jane adds the kick and boldness to our recipes and to our life. We are lucky to live next door to her; her husband, Brian; and their three children. We find it endlessly exciting to test new recipes, and it's so easy to run back and forth with something new to try.

Jane presents at conferences, retreats, and immersions both on her own and with my husband and me. We travel across the country and overseas to participate in conferences, retreats, and immersions. We share with our audiences the tips and tricks we've learned from years of cooking delicious plant-based, oil-free meals. We teach people how to get away from processed food, even if it's labeled "vegan," since it's often full of oil. We introduce them to the wonders of kale and other hearty and delicious greens, as well as sweet potatoes, artichokes, beets, broccoli, cucumbers, asparagus, whole grains, cannellini beans, lentils, and so much more.

There is no question that those patients who are the most compliant have the best results. Fortunately, it is not hard to be compliant because eating whole food, plant-based nutrition is not complicated! There is no counting anything. There are few hard-to-find products. Stick to the outside aisles of the grocery store and the produce section. Shop at farmers' markets or start your own garden. We have not included the calories or fat, protein, or carbohydrate content of the recipes on purpose. We want you to enjoy the food and not calculate anything except your blessings for having discovered the beauty of eating plant-based!

A LIFE-CHANGING STORY

"I'm a forty-five-year-old man and I've always worked out and remained active. About a year ago, however, I was experiencing chest pains. I went to see my doctor, and the results were not good: My cholesterol was at 236; my blood pressure was creeping up; and my lipids were in the high range. A carotid artery MRI revealed that, at forty-five, I had the arterial thickness of the average sixty-year-old man, and that I had substantial blockages, in the 85th percentile for my age.

"When I reviewed the test results with my doctor, he mentioned that most of this was genetic and he tried to put me on a statin drug. I refused because I was concerned about side effects (known and unknown). I mentioned that I had seen Dr. Esselstyn in the documentary *Forks over Knives* and that I felt this problem could be overcome if I followed his advice. My doctor actually told me there is no way to reverse heart disease or coronary artery disease and the best I could do was slow down the process with medications! I bought *Prevent and Reverse Heart Disease* and ate a completely plant-based diet: whole grains, veggies, and lots of beans! I stopped eating oils and processed foods as well. I also continued to work out.

"I went back to my doctor after ninety days and took another blood panel. My cholesterol had dropped to 156, my blood pressure was down to $98/60$, my lipids were low, and I wasn't having chest pains! My doctor seemed satisfied with the results—but to my dismay, he still wanted to put me on a statin drug! I told him no way and that I'd be back in a year to retake the carotid artery MRI.

"I continued with the diet for the next year, and all cravings for meat and fat went away, just as Dr. Esselstyn indicated (meat actually repulses me now). Almost one year to the day after taking the initial carotid exam, I took another and the results floored my doctor! My arterial thickness had dropped substantially. I now have the arterial thickness of the average thirty-five-year-old man, and I am in the 32nd percentile of blockages for my age group! I have aged chronologically by one year since my last test but have physiologically become many years younger. At my most recent appointment, my doctor stopped suggesting the statin drugs and advised me to keep doing whatever I'm doing."

—BILL C.

We've been bursting with new recipes since *Prevent and Reverse Heart Disease* was published, and we've been waiting anxiously to write this book. There are endless plant-based cookbooks and recipes available online these days; the problem is that they are not all safe for heart patients. So many recipes use oil, nuts (that ⅔ cup of cashews!), avocado, coconut, salt, or lots of added sugar. This cookbook is full of recipes that are scientifically proven to heal heart disease. If you take meat, dairy, and oil out of your diet, your body cannot lay down the foundation of vascular disease by injuring the innermost lining of your arteries.

Both Jane and I have been working moms with families to feed, so we know cooking often happens quickly in that snippet of time before dinner. In this cookbook, we've included some simple recipes such as one-bowl, delicious and hearty rice-and-beans meals, which are our go-to weekday dinners. Fast Pasta and Greens (page 238) and Five-Star Rice and Beans (page 206) make satisfying meals during the week, too. But you'll also find some inventive surprises like Nori Noir (page 216), Carrot Dogs (page 67), Philly-Style Soft Pretzels (page 144), our signature "Enlightened" Dr. Seuss Stacked Polenta (page 130), and Jane's out-of-this world Kale Cake with Blueberry Frosting (page 256).

The third paragraph of the Greek Hippocratic oath reads: "I will use those dietary regimens which will benefit my patients according to my greatest ability and adjustment, and I will do no harm or injustice to them." And yet, in spite of all the evidence-based research on patients reversing their disease through a plant-based diet—not only my husband's research but research performed by Dr. John McDougall, Dr. Neal Barnard, Dr. Dean Ornish, and T. Colin Campbell, PhD, at Cornell—most cardiologists do not offer a plant-based diet as a preventative measure to patients because they say the patients won't comply.

What we've seen, time and again, is exactly the opposite. Thanks to the success of *Prevent and Reverse Heart Disease* and the blockbuster documentary *Forks over Knives*, which featured my husband and T. Colin Campbell and their pioneering research, the message is getting to the public. A growing number of politicians, actors, producers, and television hosts are changing their diets.

Sometimes people ask how our family can sustain eating as we do. Our answer consists of four reasons: It is simple, it tastes good, we feel wonderful, and we know we are maximally protected from chronic illness. This book is not just a collection of recipes—it is a collection of wisdom around a lifestyle of cooking, family, and health.

Truly, the biggest gift my husband and I have given our children and grandchildren is the joy of whole food, plant-based eating. We hope this cookbook will bring that joy to you and your loved ones and that you will discover, as one patient did, that "This program is an anchor in the midst of a raging sea of ideas that don't really work. I feel planted as I maintain its regimen." May you, too, be anchored in the joy of whole food, plant-based eating.

—**Ann Crile Esselstyn and Jane Esselstyn**

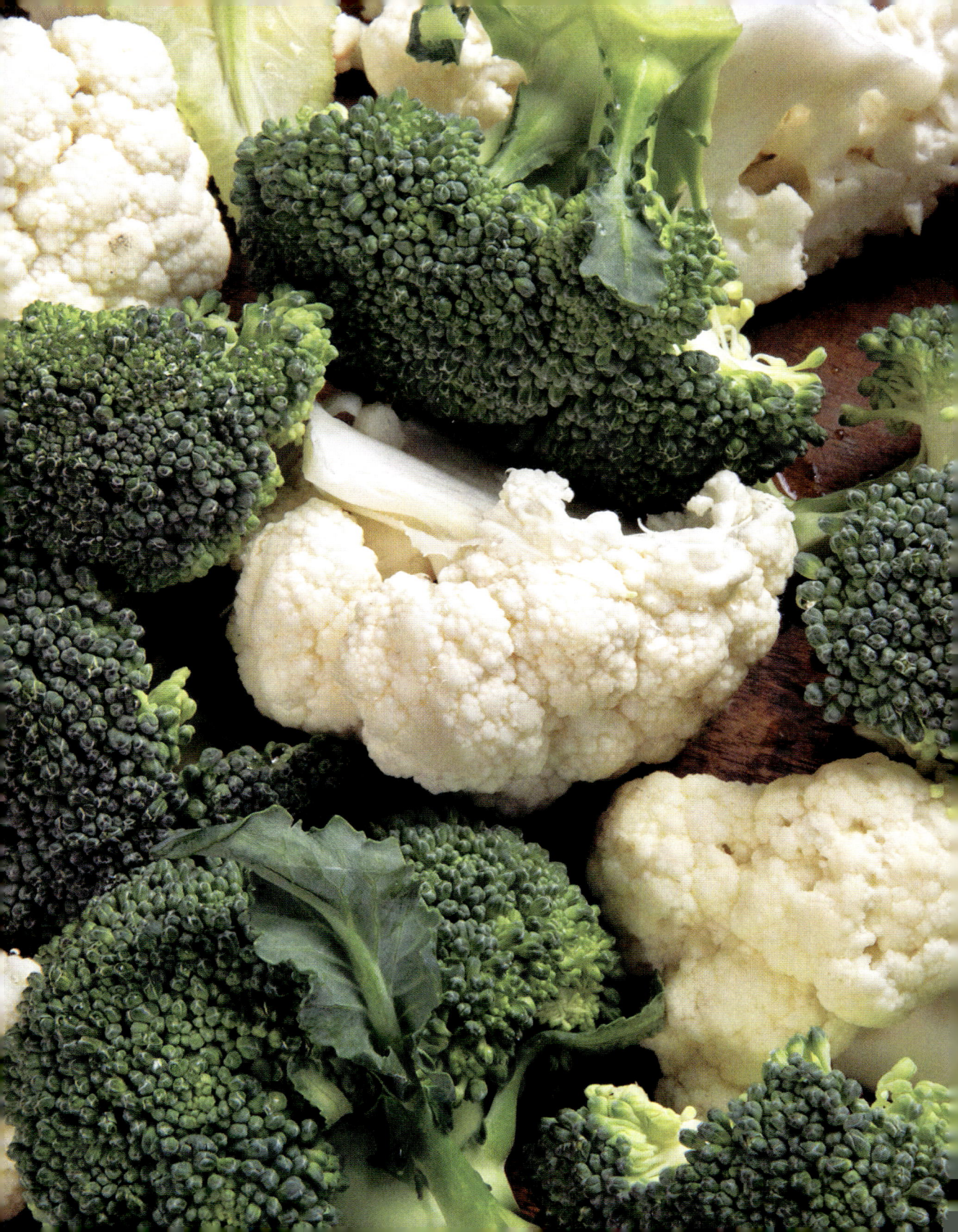

GETTING STARTED IN YOUR *PREVENT AND REVERSE HEART DISEASE* KITCHEN

When you are making a change in the way you eat, we know it can feel overwhelming. This chapter will walk you through the very simple, practical ways you can ready your pantry and your kitchen for easy, everyday cooking the *Prevent and Reverse Heart Disease* way. But first, here's our 12-step program to help you get over any hurdles and to make the nutritional guidelines of the program simple. It's all you need to remember.

OUR 12-STEP PROGRAM FOR PLANT-PERFECT EATING

1. Eat no meat, pork, fish, or fowl. No flesh. None. Every cell in an animal is made of cholesterol. All meat also has saturated fat and animal protein. And new research suggests that digesting meat releases a by-product, trimethylamine N-oxide (TMAO), an even stronger predictor of heart disease than cholesterol. *Avoid* highly processed fake vegan and soy "meats" because they have a lot of oil in them.

2. Consume no dairy products. Like meat, all dairy products contain cholesterol, saturated fat, animal protein, and casein. The protein in dairy is one of the most relevant carcinogens identified. *Avoid* all highly processed vegan and soy cheeses, which are made with a lot of oil and often have added casein!

3. Eliminate oil! All oil. Get rid of all the oil in your cupboards, even if it's virgin olive oil, so that you *can't* use it. Instead of using oil when you stir-fry and sauté vegetables, you can use vegetable broth (no sodium added), water, wine, beer, or vinegar. They all work well. Instead of relying on oil when you bake, use applesauce, apple butter without sugar, pureed prunes, or mashed ripe bananas. We'll help you create an oil-free salad dressing you'll *love* (see pages 167–79) and soon you will never miss the oil-filled ones. Balsamic vinegars are delicious on salad and the flavor-infused ones are stunningly good.

4. Eat whole-grain oats. Old-fashioned rolled oats or steel-cut oats are good choices. Avoid the more processed "quick-cooking" or "instant" oats. Oats help lower cholesterol and blood sugar, reduce artery inflammation, and are dose-responsive, so find a breakfast with oats you love, then eat oats, in some fashion, *every day*! Enjoy whole-grain oats for breakfast any way you can—either as oatmeal or as a cold cereal with non-dairy milk and fruit, or in the batter for waffles or pancakes.

5. Eat whole grains. Be sure the word *whole* is in front of wheat or rye in the ingredient list. And be sure the word *brown* is in front of rice. If you don't see "whole" in front of the grain on a bread label, it's likely made with white flour fancied up to sound impressive. (Also check to be sure that there is no added oil in bread products.) Many wonderful whole-grain products are available in the cooler section and the frozen food aisle.

6. Eat greens, especially leafy greens, as well as all the symphony of rainbow-colored vegetables. Cooked or raw, vegetables are king! Make leafy greens—like kale, collards, and Swiss chard—the nest on which you put your food; mix greens directly into your food; or pile greens on the side of your plate. Mix greens into soup. If you're making pasta, add small pieces of kale or other leafy greens to the pot four minutes before the pasta is done then drain the whole pot, and you have a meal in one. Make kale sandwiches. Use collard leaves instead of burritos in a wrap. Roll up a collard green like a sushi roll. Mix a bunch of greens into pasta sauce and spread it on your whole wheat, no-oil pizza crust, then top with veggies—but, of course, *no* cheese.

7. Eat beans and lentils! All beans and lentils are delicious and filling and are healthy protein sources. Try red lentils in soup. They cook quickly and give the soup a nice color. Put beans in salads. Hummus, which must be made without tahini or oil, has become our "mayonnaise" for spreading on sandwiches and is our favorite dip for vegetables and crackers. It's even an ingredient in our favorite salad dressing. Our main party dish is brown rice and black beans piled high with chopped tomatoes, thawed frozen corn, chopped green onions, water chestnuts, cilantro, chopped arugula, chopped peppers, etc., and topped with salsa.

8. Avoid sugar as much as possible. Always avoid drinking fruit juice. Eat the whole fruit instead. Read labels and avoid added sugars. Don't get caught up thinking one sugar is better than another. Avoid them all as much as possible. Save sweets for birthdays or special holiday treats. Instead put grapes in your freezer for an amazing sweet treat or freeze bananas or mangoes and blend them in a high-speed blender or a Yonanas machine for delicious dairy-free "ice cream." Also, a little fruit or dried fruit added to a dish can really help sweeten it up. We use pure maple syrup in some recipes because it has the least amount of fructose of all sweeteners.

9. Avoid salt as much as possible. Look at the government label for the amount of salt (sodium) in a product. No added salt is ideal, or aim for the salt content being equal to the calorie content or less. Instead of salt, add vinegar, lemon juice, lime juice, or low-sodium hot sauces for flavor. You will lose your taste for salt before you know it. Gourmet salts like Celtic salt and sea salt are no better. Don't get caught up thinking one is better than another. Avoid them all as much as possible.

10. Steer clear of nuts, avocado, and coconut. Instead, use 1 to 2 tablespoons of ground flaxseeds or chia seeds daily on cereal or in salads—both are excellent for omega-3 fatty acids. An occasional sprinkling of sesame seeds is fine.

11. Drink water! You can't go wrong with water. You will save thousands of dollars and thousands of calories by just drinking water. Absolutely never drink sodas, artificially sweetened or not. Avoid smoothies. Don't drink your calories; chew them. You can flavor water; soda water; or seltzer water with slices of orange, lemon or lime, or splash of orange or apple juice occasionally but never drink juice by the glass on a regular basis!

12. Read food labels, especially the ingredients. You will be surprised how often products that claim to have "zero fat" will list oil among their ingredients. The government allows anything under 0.5 grams of fat to be labeled *fat free*. Even products labeled *trans fat free* can have trans fat in them if you see partially hydrogenated oil as an ingredient! Shocking. Be vigilant!

Sometimes a simple ingredient you've never heard of can be a speed bump that thwarts your enthusiasm. But fear not! March forth and be the champion of your own health. The following pages contain some go-to basics we like to have on hand. Some are ingredients and some are products. They'll help you stock your pantry so that you are ready to dive right in to the recipes later in the book.

Nutritional Yeast

We always have nutritional yeast around. It is *very* different from what people think of as yeast. Nutritional yeast is dry, flaky, and pale yellow in color, and it is often found in the bulk section of health food stores or occasionally prepackaged on the grocery store shelf. It is a great source of protein and has a nice nutty, creamy flavor. We use it the way others use Parmesan cheese—it adds extra flavor and a creamier texture when melted into or sprinkled on a dish.

Balsamic Vinegars

Our arsenal is stacked with vinegars, ones we find, ones we special order, ones we are given, and ones that are our go-to everyday workhorses. Vinegar does an excellent job of enhancing taste when you are cooking without salt. There are many different balsamic vinegar stores across the country. We were first introduced to the magic of infused vinegars by a company called the Olive Tap (www.olivetap.com). Since then, we have found other excellent sources for infused vinegars including a store called Bema and Pa's (bemaandpas.com) located in Chicago and Olio2go (olio2go.com) for a wonderful white balsamic vinegar, Acetaia Cattani White Balsamic Vinegar. White balsamic is a good choice when you don't want the dark color of traditional balsamic

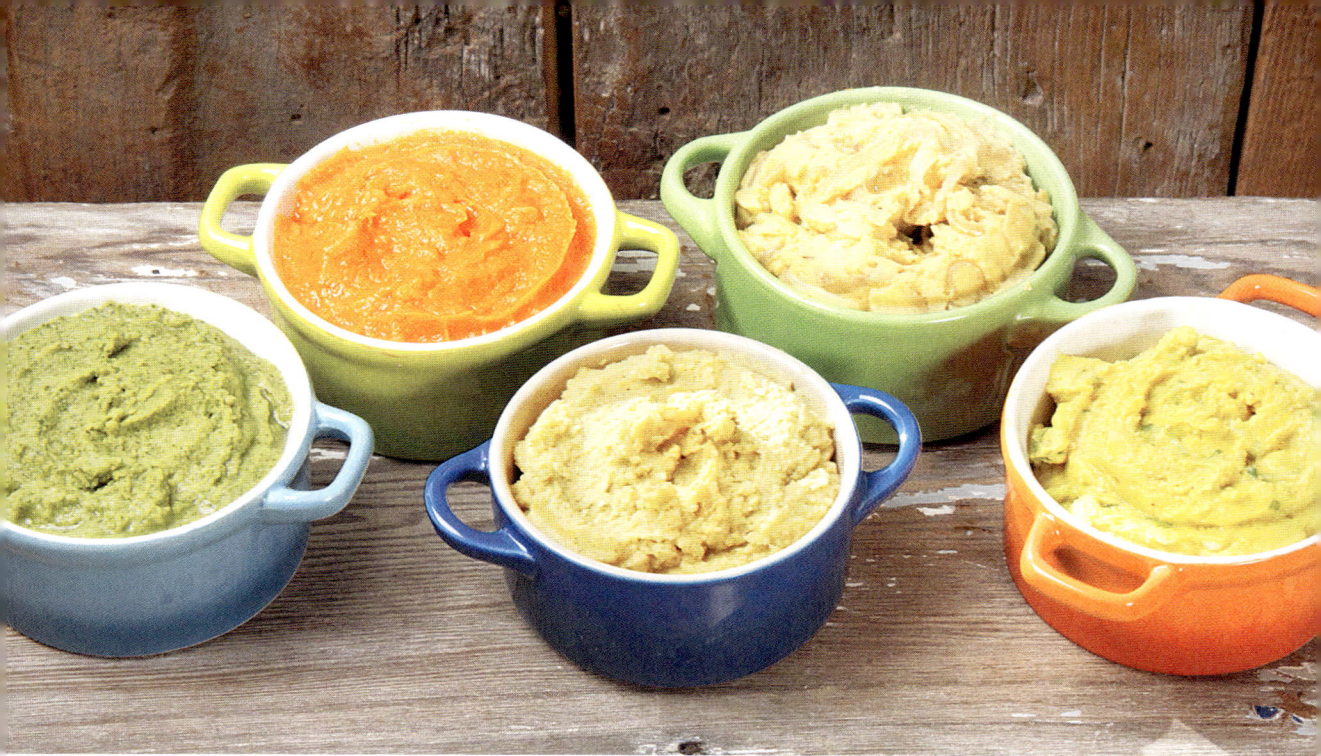

vinegars. It works well with Cauliflower Steaks (page 233) and Oberlin Corn and Shallot Chowder (page 89). It's a lot of fun to find a store specializing in vinegars and to taste the amazing variety. But you don't need high-end or infused vinegar for everyday use. A great basic balsamic vinegar is a big bottle of Kirkland brand from Costco.

Hummus

Hummus without any added tahini or oil has become our new mayonnaise, and we use it as a sandwich spread, favorite dip, and as the base of different salad dressings and so many other recipes. It is easy to make your own, so we offer a number of varieties in this book: Our Hummus (page 102), Caramelized Onion Hummus (page 104), Sweet Potato Hummus (page 105), Green Onion Hummus (page 103), and Pesto Hummus (page 106). It is also convenient to buy hummus. All Whole Foods Market stores carry Engine 2 brand no-added-tahini or -oil hummus, in a variety of flavors. Oasis, Sahara Cuisine, and Amir are available in a number of grocery stores in no-added-tahini or -oil varieties as well.

Tofu

Tofu has a high fat content, so we use it sparingly and mostly in desserts. It's essential to use the proper type of tofu in some dessert recipes to ensure you get a smooth yet firm texture. We use silken lite firm tofu by Mori-Nu. Regular tofu is grainier in texture and some smooth tofu is runny like yogurt. We use neither type in this book.

Flaxseed Meal and Chia Seeds

Eat flaxseed meal or chia seeds daily sprinkled on cereal or in salads to supply omega-3 fatty acids. Flaxseeds need to be ground before consumption and should always be kept refrigerated or frozen after being ground. Chia seeds do not need to be ground or refrigerated. Both also work as thickeners. As an egg substitute, combine 1 tablespoon flaxseed meal and 3 tablespoons water, or 1 tablespoon chia seeds and ¼ cup water, to replace 1 egg.

Bread and Flour

Ezekiel bread by the Food for Life brand is made with sprouted grains and contains no added oil. It is widely available (often in the frozen food section) from Whole Foods, Trader Joe's, health food stores, and many local grocery stores. The bread comes in low-sodium, sesame, and cinnamon-raisin flavors. There are also English muffins, tortillas, burger buns, and hot dog buns. There are other good breads. Just always read the labels. Our favorite pizza crust is Sami's Millet and Flax Pizza Crust. We often order five at a time online from Samisbakery.com.

We use four kinds of flour in this book: white whole wheat (which is *not* a white, "all-purpose" flour but rather flour made from white wheat berries), barley, chickpea, and oat bran flour. Feel free to use the 100 percent whole-grain flour of your choice.

Nondairy Milk

There are many nondairy milks; find the one that suits you best. We recommend unsweetened almond milk or oat milk. Nonfat soy milk is available, but beware of added sugar. We do not recommend rice milk, as it contains added oil.

Vegetable Broth

We use vegetable broth in many dishes and it can also be a great liquid to use to stir-fry and sauté vegetables instead of oil. What's best, when you have the time, is to make your own broth with the ends of vegetables and leftover vegetable cooking liquid. But you can absolutely buy good vegetable broth at the grocery store—just go with a lower-sodium brand. We like Kitchen Basics, which is widely available. It is dark in color, however, so when we make dishes in which color is important, we use a lighter broth like Pacific Organic low sodium brand. Here are a few options:

- Kitchen Basics Unsalted Vegetable Cooking Stock (240 mg sodium per cup). The only sodium comes from the vegetables—no salt is added to the stock itself.
- Pacific Organic Fat-Free Low-Sodium Vegetable Broth (140 mg sodium per cup)
- Health Valley Fat-Free Vegetable Broth (360 mg sodium per cup)

Others exist. Just read the ingredients and check the sodium content, and when you can't find what you want, make your own.

Beans and Lentils

Beans canned or dried are excellent. Be aware of the sodium content in canned beans. Whole Foods 365 beans are salt free and 89¢ a can, hard to beat unless you make your own from dried beans. Just always read ingredients and sodium content. If the beans have sodium, be sure to drain and rinse them. Eden organic makes salt-free, BPA-free beans, but they are expensive.

There are many different kinds of lentils. Use them all. Red lentils dissolve quickly and give soup a good color. Green and black lentils keep their shape and work well in salads.

Engine 2 Products

Whole Foods carries a number of Engine 2 products that are low-sodium, low-sugar, 100 percent plant-based and 100 percent whole-grain with no meat, dairy, or added oil. Engine 2 hummus (which contains some sesame seeds, which is fine), veggie burgers, frozen grains, almond milk, crackers, pasta sauce, sprouted grain, and brown rice tortillas all follow the *Prevent and Reverse* guidelines. Look for more products coming all the time.

Sweeteners

The only sweetener we use besides fruit is 100 percent pure maple syrup. The good news is that it is delicious—the bad news is, it's expensive. We use it sparingly in some places and more prominently as a sweetener in other recipes. Do not use any cheap imitations as they are filled with unhealthy ingredients. Also avoid artificial sweeteners. They simply help maintain that urge for sweetness. *Taste changes!* Have faith.

Greens: Kale, Collards, Swiss Chard, Etc.

You can cut up leafy greens and add them to anything for a big nutritional boost. Don't be intimidated by greens like kale and collards. They are both delicious green powerhouses! Both kale and collards, as well as some other greens, have tough central spines that we strip off. Do not balk at this—stripping actually makes the preparation fast and fun and turns kale into "spinach with heft."

To strip kale or collards, hold the end of the stem firmly with one hand. Wrap your other hand just below the leafy part. Gently but firmly slide your hand up the leaf, staying close to the stem to strip off the leaf. You may discard the stems, or, as we often do, cut them on an angle and add them to soups or cook them until tender and add them to salads. Our dog loves them, too. To chop the leaves, cut them into strips with a knife and then cut them again crosswise; alternatively, you can cut them using kitchen shears, or just tear them into pieces with your hands. We also often cook the leaves whole, then cut them in the colander when we're draining them or right in the pot with kitchen shears.

Many greens do not have tough certral spines and don't need to be stripped or chopped in order to eat. Beet greens, Swiss chard, mustard greens, bok choy, and spinach are less dense than kale or collards and thus require less prep and cooking time to become tender.

You definitely don't need a lot of fancy equipment to cook plant-based, oil-free meals. But there are a few tools in our kitchen that we love:

- **Rice cooker**—A rice cooker is helpful for cooking rice or other grains. Just follow the directions for the grain and add the correct amount of water (or broth), and the rice cooker takes care of the cooking. We use our rice cooker for brown rice, quinoa, barley, couscous, farro—all our grains.

- **Microplane**—This terrific gadget is great for zesting! Limes, lemons, and oranges have so much to offer in their rinds. Zesting them is an easy and fun way to get more flavor without too much citrus.

- **Citrus reamer**—While a Microplane is perfect for removing citrus *zest*, a citrus reamer is great for removing the juice. This is especially good with limes. We love the wooden ones.

- **Lemon squeezer**—A lemon squeezer or press is another way to remove all the juice from lemons and limes. It also catches all the lemon seeds, which is a huge help. (FYI, limes do not have seeds!)

- **Food processor**—A food processor will shred, grate, slice, and mix hard and soft foods. It is an invaluable kitchen addition, and a good one does not need to be expensive.

- **Immersion blender**—An immersion blender is a time-saving help because you can put it right in the soup pot and blend. We love how it decreases the dirty dishes.

- **Perfect Tortilla or tortilla bowl makers**—These little pans form sturdy, crispy bowls out of whole-grain or rice tortillas; see Crispy Tortilla Bowls recipe (page 30).

- **Yonanas machine or Dessert Bullet**—These pieces of equipment are not essential, but if you have one you can make the healthiest, most delicious, all-fruit frozen desserts. The Yonanas machine is widely available and not too expensive. It works best with bananas as the base ingredient. The Dessert Bullet is more expensive but allows you to use other fruits to make nondairy "ice cream." See our recipe for Banana Soft Serve (page 264).

- **Parchment paper**—This is a lifesaver, especially because we do not use oil or cooking spray. We use parchment paper to line everything from baking sheets to lasagna pans to cake pans to avoid sticking and a messy cleanup.

These are the recipes you'll return to again and again: when you are making complex dishes, when enjoying on their own, or when using as toppings (we like to have a supply of the roasted red peppers around all the time!).

COOKED KALE

SERVES 5 TO 6

There are as many ways to eat kale, collards, and other greens as there are those of us eating them. Kale is spectacularly beautiful and oh so delicious! We have found guests always love kale this simple way, even when they are not kale aficionados. This recipe works equally well for collards; in fact, we often mix the two together. You can also follow this method if you are cooking Swiss chard, in which case you do not need to cook it as long or remove the stems—they are edible.

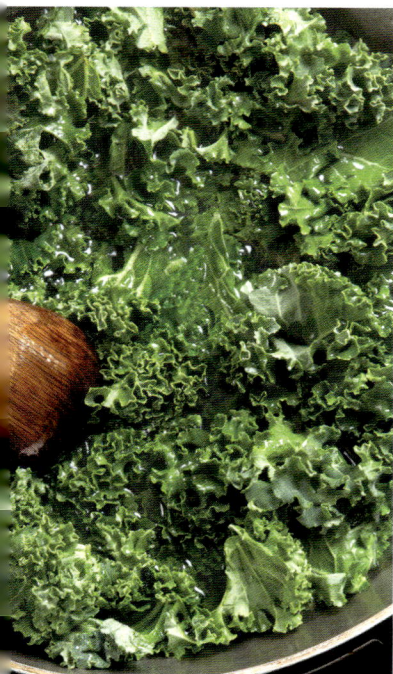

INGREDIENTS:

2 bunches kale, stems stripped and leaves torn in bite-size pieces

INSTRUCTIONS:

Bring a large pot of water to a boil. Place the kale leaves in the water, cover, and cook until tender, about 5 minutes. Drain in a colander.

Serve warm, alone or with Sweet Corn Sauce (page 111), Lemony Cheezy Sauce (page 112), any of our dressings, or with nice balsamic vinegars!

ROASTED RED PEPPERS

These are luscious! We add them to salads, salad dressings, sandwiches, wraps, rice, grains, greens, burgers, and beans. They make everything more sophisticated and yummy. We always double the recipe when we make them—if you decide to double the recipe, use the same quantities for the herbs as you would for a single batch. If you save the juice from the peppers as you roast them, it adds a feel of oil in salad dressings. It is easiest to save the juice by cooling the peppers, pricking them before peeling, and keeping the juice in the bowl with the peppers.

INGREDIENTS:

6 red bell peppers

3 tablespoons balsamic vinegar

2 teaspoons minced garlic

1 teaspoon dried basil

1 teaspoon dried thyme

1 teaspoon dried rosemary

1 teaspoon dried marjoram

1 teaspoon dried oregano

INSTRUCTIONS:

Preheat the oven to 450°F, or heat the broiler.

Place the peppers on a baking sheet and roast or broil until the skin is blackened on one side. Rotate the peppers and continue rotating and rotating until all sides are blackened. Some people prefer to roast the peppers individually over a gas flame, which also works. Remove the peppers from the oven and set aside until cool enough to handle.

Peel the skin from the roasted peppers. Slice or tear the pepper flesh into long strips and place them in a bowl. Add the vinegar, garlic, basil, thyme, rosemary, marjoram, and oregano. Allow the peppers and spices to marinate for at least 30 minutes.

Tip: Mix some of the juice from the peppers with no-tahini hummus, balsamic vinegar, mustard, and a little orange juice for a knockout salad dressing!

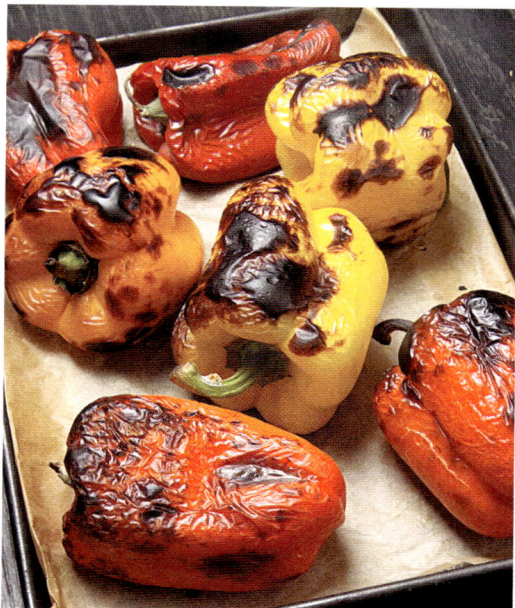
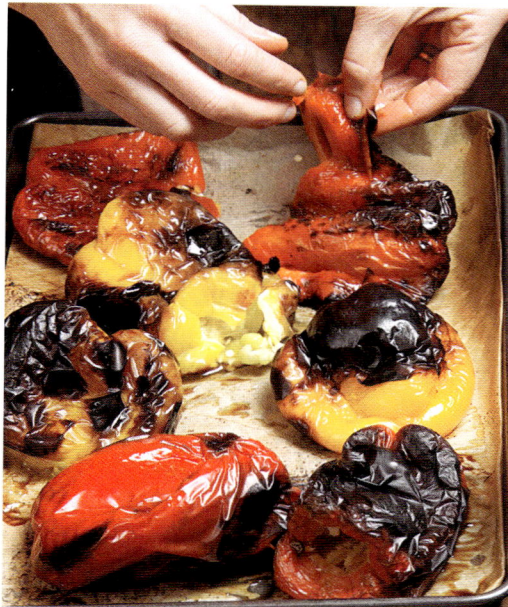
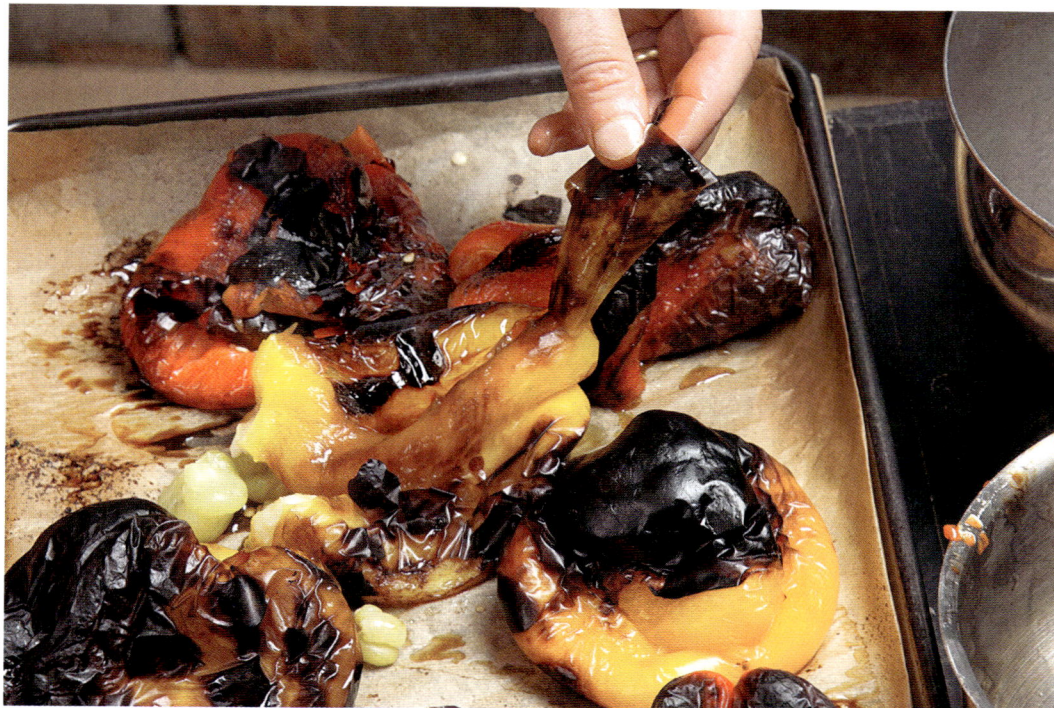

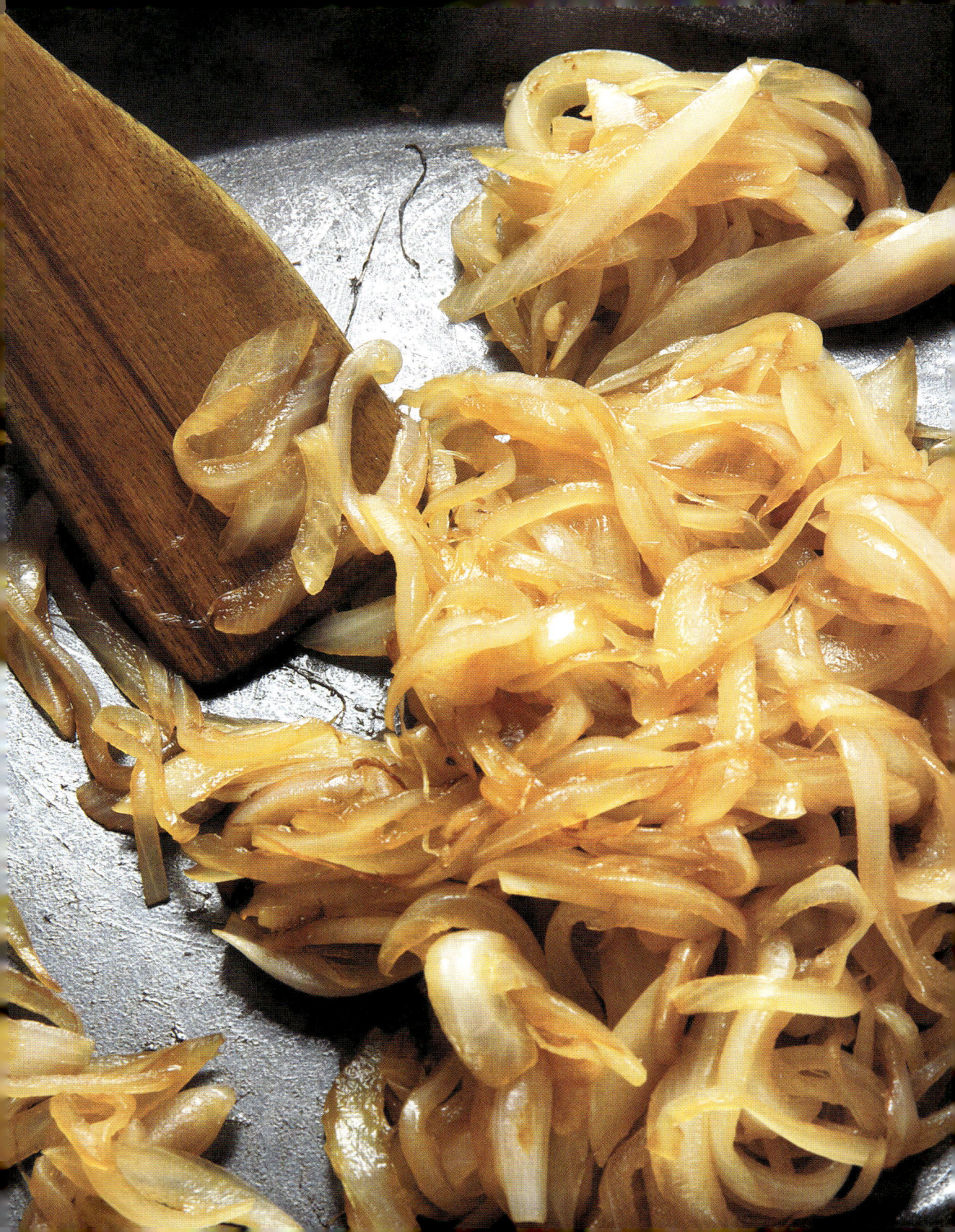

CARAMELIZED ONIONS

A hot, hot pan is the key to caramelizing onions. These are such a staple in our kitchens!

INGREDIENTS:

1 large onion, diced or julienned

INSTRUCTIONS:

Heat a frying pan over high heat. When the pan is hot enough that a drop of water does not turn to steam when dropped in the pan but rather beads around like a pearl on the surface, add the onions. Cook, stirring, until they start to brown. As you continue cooking, slowly reduce the heat. Add a teaspoon of water and continue stirring until the onions are browned and cooked through.

Serve warm or store in an airtight container in the refrigerator until ready to use.

VARIATION:

Add 1 to 2 tablespoons balsamic vinegar to the onions as they cook and stir until they are uniformly coated, and you'll have Caramelized Balsamic Onions.

SAUTÉED MUSHROOMS

We could each eat a batch of these alone every time we make them—we just love them!

INGREDIENTS:

8 ounces mushrooms, sliced

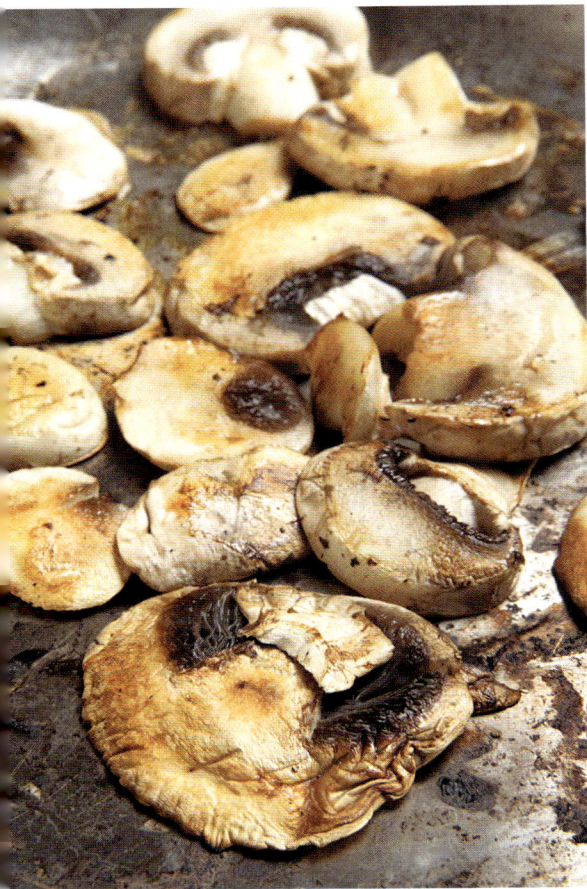

INSTRUCTIONS:

Heat a frying pan over high heat. Place the sliced mushrooms flat in the pan. No mushroom should be resting on any other mushroom—all surfaces should be in contact with the heated pan. Let them be for a minute as they start to cook; then reduce the heat to medium. Really, let them be. In a few minutes you will see them starting to brown and get fragrant.

After 4 to 5 minutes, turn them over and brown the other side. Add a little water if needed—otherwise, stir the mushrooms around in their own juices and cook for 2 minutes more.

Serve warm, or store in an airtight container in the refrigerator until ready to use.

VARIATIONS:

Add 1 tablespoon balsamic vinegar to the mushrooms just before turning and stir until they are uniformly coated, and you'll have Sautéed Balsamic Mushrooms.

Add 1 or 2 tablespoons of barbecue sauce to the mushrooms toward the end of cooking.

GRILLED PINEAPPLE

These sweet golden rings add flavor, color, and swing to any sandwich, burger, burrito, or pizza and are great on their own as a dessert!

INGREDIENTS:

1 pineapple, peeled, cored, and cut into 1-inch-thick rounds

INSTRUCTIONS:

Preheat a panini press or similar sandwich-grilling device to high heat, or heat an outdoor grill to high heat. Place the pineapple rounds on the press or grill and close the lid. Cook until dark brown grill marks appear.

Serve immediately on a Beet Burger with Grilled Pineapple (page 228) or a Dagwood Sandwich (page 65), add to a Salad Pizza (page 201), use in a salad, or just eat as a luscious treat!

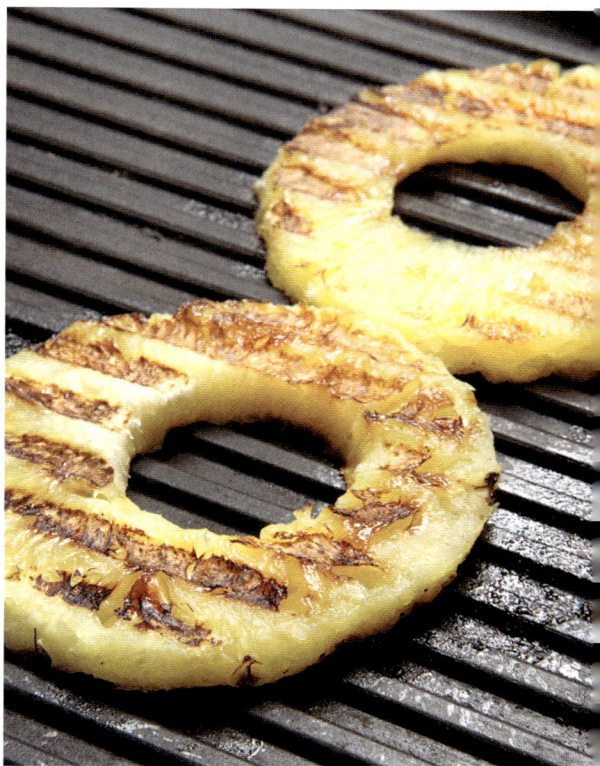

CRISPY TORTILLA BOWLS

I found tortilla bowl makers at Bed Bath & Beyond one Christmas for my mom. It happened to be the same month that Rip's Engine 2 Ancient Grains Tortillas came out at Whole Foods, so for Christmas dinner we feasted on Fire Brigade Chili from My Beef with Meat *in Crispy Tortilla Bowls made out of Rip's wraps. The bowls don't leak! Try them with Sandra's Chili (page 194) or with Sloppy Joes or Tidy Janes (page 230). You can also really impress—and make a heartier meal—by serving salads in these (see Hearty Salads chapter).*

INGREDIENTS:

  6 tortillas

INSTRUCTIONS:

Preheat the oven to 350°F.

Place the tortillas in a mold, such as a tortilla bowl maker. Bake the tortillas for 8 to 10 minutes, or until crispy from top to bottom.

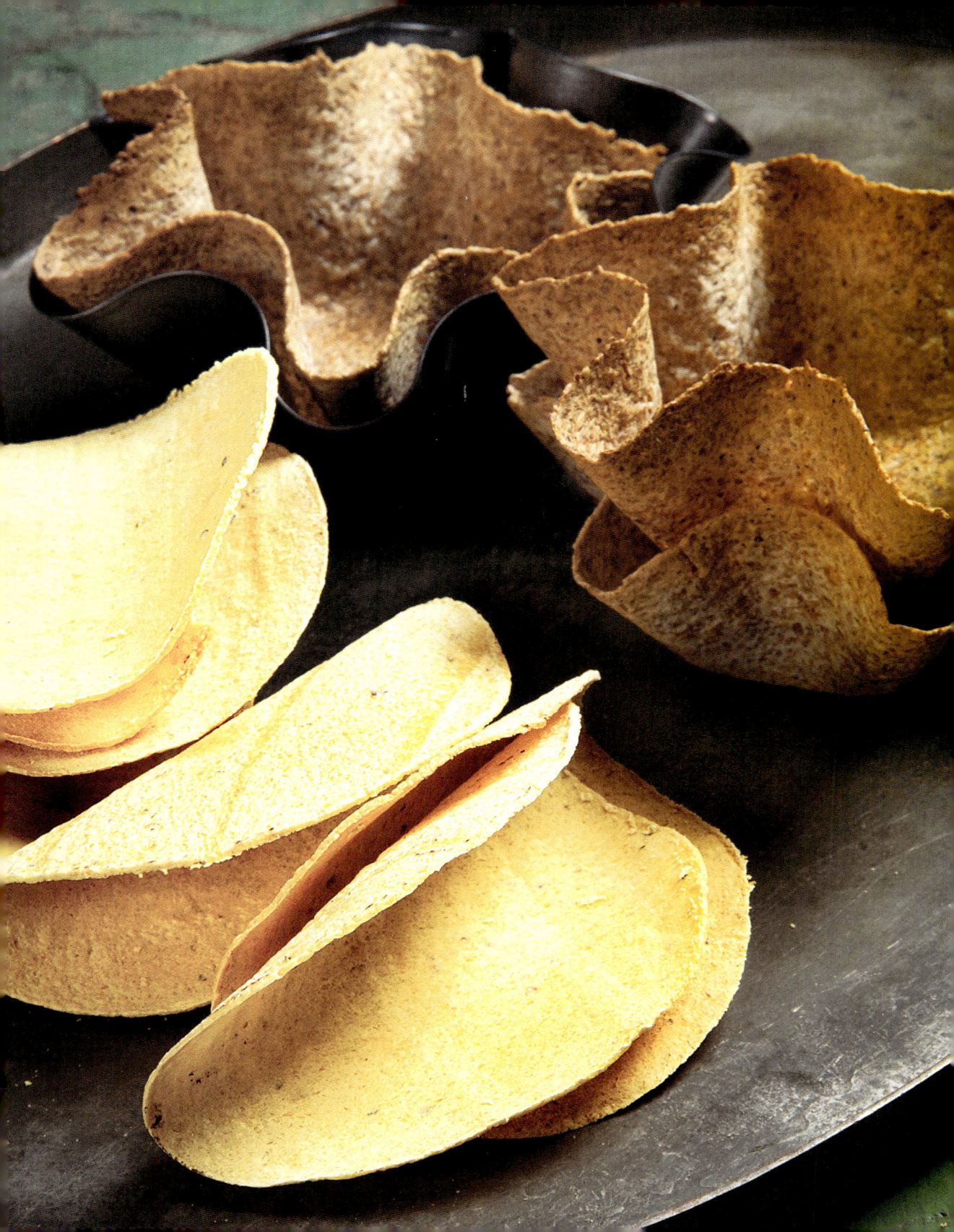

CORN TORTILLA TACO SHELLS AND TOSTADOS

We make our own taco shells or tostados from the small corn tortillas available in the dairy (gasp!) section of grocery stores. They are oil-free. They can be used to make:

- taco-shaped shells
- tostado style—flat and crispy
- tostado-chip style—broken in pieces

INGREDIENTS:

1 package corn tortillas, usually contains 10 tortillas

INSTRUCTIONS:

*Please note the photograph of the tacos and tostados on page 31 for a visual reference.

Preheat the oven to 350°F.

For taco shells, drape one tortilla over two slats of oven rack, allowing the rounded sides to hang down. Repeat for as many taco shells as you desire.

For tostados (flat, crispy tortilla rounds), lay the number of desired tortillas flat on the oven rack.

Cook in oven for 5 to 10 minutes, checking occasionally as they may burn and oven temperatures vary. Remove from oven when they are crisp. As they cool a bit, they get even crispier—serve while still warm.

A Q&A WITH DR. CALDWELL ESSELSTYN JR., MD

1. How is your approach to treating heart disease unique? My program addresses the cause of the illness, not the symptom. This program is a nutrition-based therapy that has been scientifically proven to reverse heart disease. There is no other treatment plan backed by a study as long as the one I conducted, or a study that has produced such dramatic, visible results. Coronary angiograms (X-rays) of the patients in my study show an actual reversal of the disease. To experience these benefits, my patients must strictly adhere to my plant-based diet program, but the effects are more than worth the effort. For those people who are very sick, it is the most effective treatment option—far less dangerous and more effective than invasive surgical procedures such as stents and bypass (except in acute emergencies), and much more effective than drugs alone. Traditional cardiology has relied on technology to ease the symptoms of heart disease but has not addressed its causes. My approach is not another stopgap solution; it prevents heart disease from occurring in those who don't yet have the disease, and it heals the body and reverses the disease when symptoms are present. Best of all, over time the benefits endure and continue to improve. I am always excited when I see arrest and reversal in patient after patient and their joy and relief when they are free of the disease that was destroying them.

2. What would you say to someone considering a stent or other surgical procedures or drug therapy to treat their heart disease? All heart patients who are not absolute emergencies should first have an aggressive opportunity at nonsurgical medical therapy. This is not just my opinion but that of expert cardiologists from Boston, Hartford, Houston, Stanford, San Diego, Seattle, and Cleveland. The difference in my case is that I advocate an aggressive plant-based nutrition program to arrest and reverse the disease and to avoid all surgery. Drugs alone do not prevent heart attacks or stop symptoms of heart disease.

3. Where should my LDL be? LDL is the "bad" cholesterol. The closer it can be to 80–85 or lower, the better. If, however, one is unable to take statin drugs and is eating plant-based nutrition, and the LDL won't go lower than 95–105, it would appear that the person will still be fine. The lesson we learned from the Tarahumara Indians, who never have cardiovascular disease, is that the most key protective element is knowing that nothing that is a building block of vascular disease or can injure endothelium is eaten.

4. Should I take statins or not? Statins are not the reason that cultures such as the Tarahumara and the Papua Highlanders do not have cardiovascular disease. Statins appear to have modest benefits in primary prevention and are of some help in slowing disease progression for those who already have an established diagnosis of cardiovascular disease. Clearly, though, some of our most profound successes in arresting and reversing disease were with patients who either refused or were incapable of taking statins. Nothing is as powerful for the prevention of cardiovascular disease as plant-based nutrition.

5. I have a family history of heart disease. Does that matter? Our data indicates that even those with strong family history of vascular disease are protected when eating a plant-based diet. Family history loads the gun, but lifestyle pulls the trigger.

A LIFE-CHANGING STORY

"I've lost fifty pounds; gone from chest discomfort almost every day to hardly ever; from left-arm pain a few times a week to almost never; from 150 mg Toprol-XL to 25 mg; from long-ago 80 mg Zocor that didn't help much to only 20 mg Crestor from a total cholesterol lifetime high of 333 to 140; took some time, but my LDL finally dropped to 80; I went from 5.5 hours of sleep a night to 8 hours, for the first time in more than twenty years; my chronic low-level sinus infection is gone, too. Almost best of all is that from about the two-month mark I suddenly felt very much better, better than I could remember feeling in decades!

> "That's my story—and all from doing such a little thing: eating what's good for me and not eating what's bad for me—what an amazing miracle!
>
> "My cardiologist is very happy—my internist got teary-eyed—we all thank Dr. Esselstyn and all of you so very much!"
>
> —SHEILA C.

6. Where do I get my protein? The protein available in a diet of whole grains, legumes, fruit, beans, and red, yellow, and green vegetables is adequate to nourish even professional athletes such as those who compete in Ironman events, professional football, mixed martial arts, and track and field. Avoid protein drinks. The extra protein is truly unnecessary and has the potential for harm if it contains animal protein.

7. Where do I get calcium? Calcium supplementation is unnecessary. There is more than adequate calcium in a plant-based diet of whole grains, legumes, and especially green leafy vegetables.

8. Why does the diet eliminate oil entirely? NO OIL! Not even olive oil—which goes against a lot of other advice out there about so-called good fats. The reality is that oils are extremely low in terms of nutritive value. They contain no fiber, no minerals, and are 100 percent fat calories. Both the monounsaturated and saturated fats contained in oils are harmful to the endothelium, the innermost lining of the arteries, and that injury is the gateway to vascular disease. It doesn't matter whether it's olive oil, corn oil, coconut oil, canola oil, or any other kind. Avoid *all* oil. This is so important that I devoted chapter 10 of my book *Prevent and Reverse Heart Disease* to oil.

9. Why should I eliminate nuts and avocado? As nuts are a rich source of saturated fats, my preference is no nuts for heart disease patients. That also eliminates peanuts and peanut butter, even though peanuts are officially a legume. For those with established heart disease, adding saturated fat from nuts is inappropriate. For people with no heart disease who want to eat nuts and avocado and are able to achieve a cholesterol of 150 and LDL of 80 or under without cholesterol-lowering drugs, some nuts

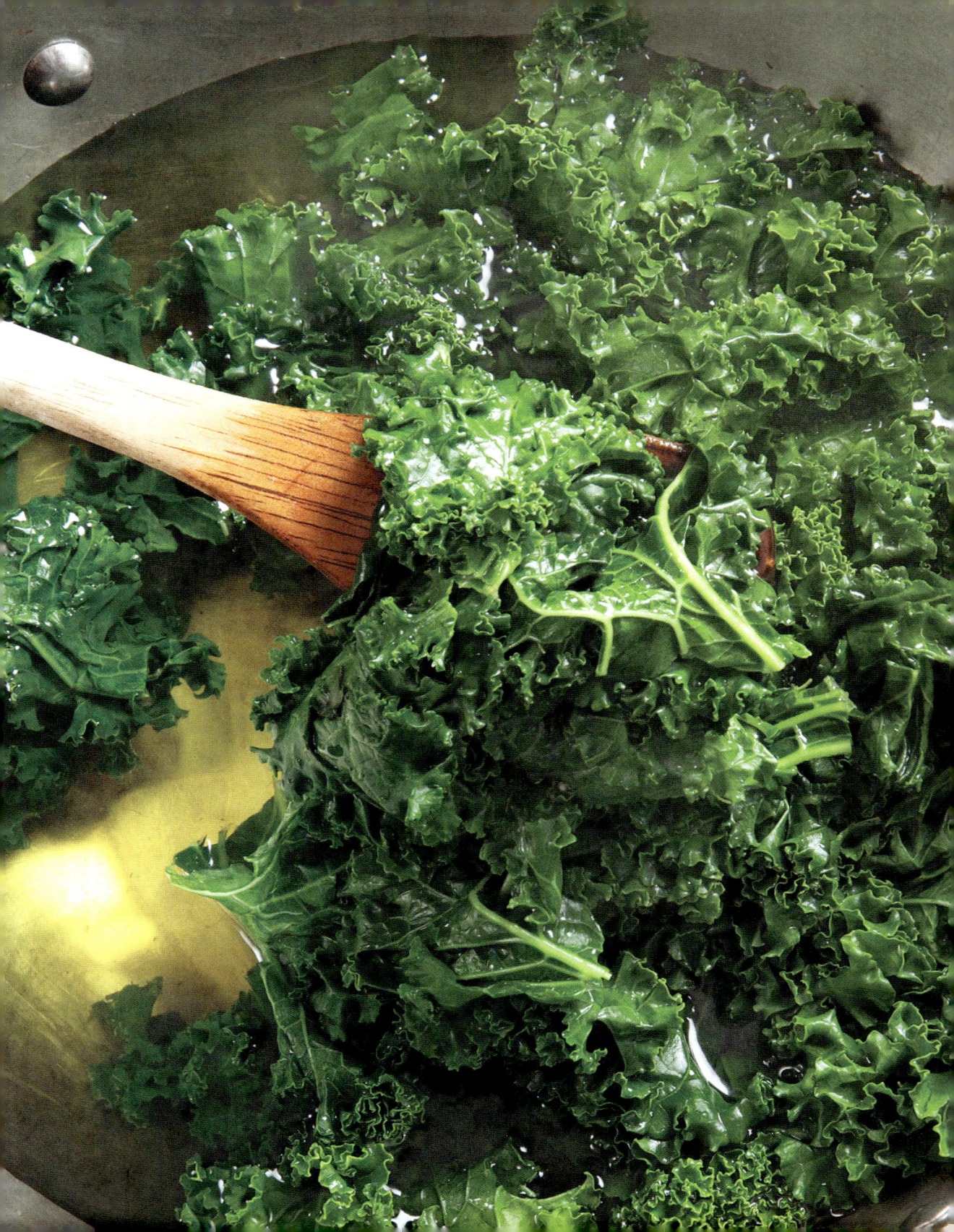

and avocado are acceptable. Chestnuts, which are very low in fat, are the one nut that are okay for those with heart disease to eat.

A LIFE-CHANGING STORY

"I am an anesthesiologist in Flagstaff, Arizona. Five years ago, I scored 1193 on a coronary artery calcium scan. I went on a plant-based diet and it was very helpful. But I still couldn't get off Crestor and Lisinopril. My LDL was still 123 off of meds! The only fats I was eating were nuts and avocado in my evening salad.

"Three months ago, I started Dr. Esselstyn's program, and the results have been nothing short of miraculous. I've lost sixteen pounds, I feel terrific, my athletic performance as a cyclist has soared. My endothelium is singing! I just got my labs back, and my cholesterol is 143 and my LDL is 78! Completely off of statins. I weaned myself off of Lisinopril, and my blood pressure is $117/74$. This is the first time in fifteen years that I've been completely off of cholesterol and blood pressure medication. The unbelievable thing is that my diet was vegan and very low fat before. What a difference a couple of handfuls of nuts and some avocado make!"

—JIM G.

10. Are seeds like flaxseeds, chia seeds, pumpkin seeds, and sesame seeds okay to eat? One to 2 tablespoons of ground flaxseeds or chia seeds daily as a source of omega-3 fatty acids are appropriate for everyone, including heart patients, if they wish. Some seeds baked in bread or crackers are acceptable. Just don't eat handfuls.

11. What is wrong with egg whites, fat-free yogurt, and skim milk, all of which have less fat? Egg whites, fat-free milk, and yogurt *all* contain animal protein, and animal protein injures the lining of the arteries. Intestinal bacteria of omnivores produces TMAO, which creates vascular injury. Do not eat even fat-free or low-fat foods containing animal protein.

12. How do I get my omega-3s? Omega-3 fatty acids are essential fatty acids supplied in adequate amounts in people consuming plant-based nutrition with plenty of leafy green vegetables. One to 2 tablespoons of ground flaxseeds or chia seeds daily, however, are perfectly acceptable to supplement this. Avoid flaxseed oil.

13. Should I take fish oil? Fish oil is not essential. Fish get their omega-3 from plants. It is difficult to be deficient in omega-3 if you are eating 1 to 2 tablespoons of ground flaxseeds or chia seeds and leafy green vegetables at several meals a day. There is also research that suggests that those on plant-based nutrition become highly efficient in manufacturing their own omega-3. Patients on fish oil are also at increased risk for bleeding, and studies now indicate that fish oil is of no benefit for heart disease patients.

14. What vitamins should I take? Take vitamin B_{12}. If you are eating copious amounts of leafy green vegetables, a multivitamin is unnecessary. Have your blood tested for vitamin D levels and supplement as appropriate to maintain blood levels in the low normal range.

15. How about smoothies? Avoid smoothies. When the fiber is pureed, it is not chewed and does not have the opportunity to mix with the facultative anaerobic bacteria that reside in the crypts and grooves of our tongues. These bacteria are capable of reducing the nitrates in green leafy vegetables to nitrates in the mouth. When the nitrates are swallowed, they are further reduced by gastric acid to nitric oxide, which may now enter the nitric oxide pool. Furthermore, chewing fruit causes the fructose to bind to the fiber, making absorption safe and slow. On the other hand, when fruit is blenderized, the fructose is separated from the fiber and the absorption is very rapid through the stomach. This rapid absorption tends to injure the liver, glycates protein, and injures the endothelial cells.

16. Is it all right to juice? Do not juice. Fructose, the sugar in fruit, is separated from fiber in juicing and is too rapidly absorbed. This is injurious. You lose the benefits of fiber, which is best obtained by eating the whole fruit or vegetable. Chew your food, especially your greens.

17. What about fruit juice? Drinking fruit juice is like pouring a sugar bowl down your throat. It is fine to eat the whole fruit. Do not drink the juice.

18. What should I drink? Water.

19. Is it all right to drink coconut water? Coconut water is 8 percent saturated fat and about 50 percent sugar. Save your money and don't buy it.

20. Can you actually enjoy food on the program? Everyone loves the food once they give it a try. It is all a matter of attitude—and you do need a positive attitude to get started and to understand that this new way of eating is the best thing you can do for your body. Then, the body will help you adjust. You actually begin to lose your physiologically-based craving for fat and sugar as their receptors in the brain become progressively reduced. Once that occurs, you can fully appreciate the natural taste of plant foods—the colorful tastes and textures are difficult to surpass.

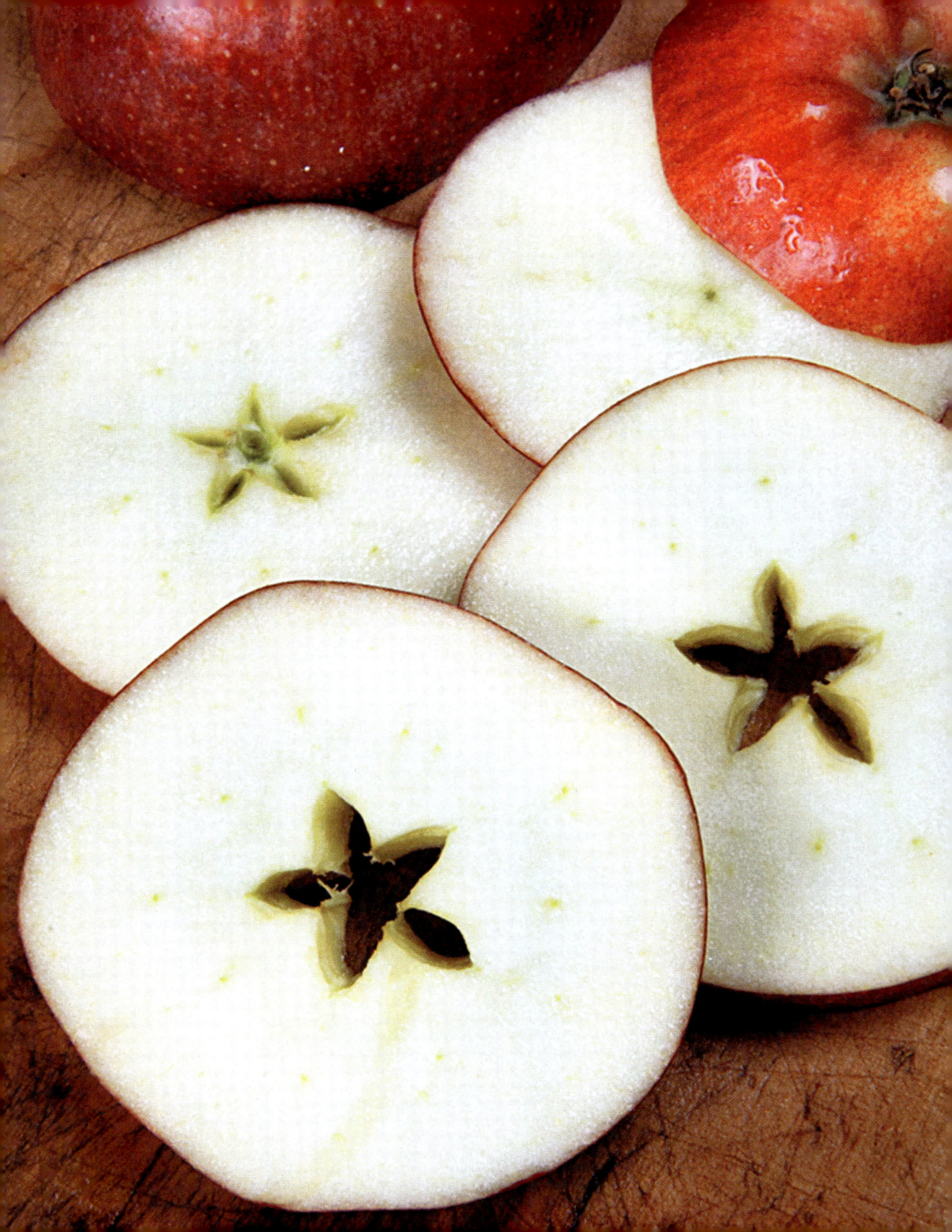

BREAKFASTS

Here's the best advice we can give you about how to start your day off right: Eat OATS! Find some way to incorporate oats into your breakfast every day. Even if you think you don't like oats, eat them. The crazy thing is, before you know it, you will like them. It is remarkable how tastes change.

THREE REASONS WHY OATS ARE IMPORTANT TO EAT DAILY:

1. Oats help lower your cholesterol.
2. Oats help decrease inflammation.
3. Oats are dose-responsive, so the more oats you eat, the more effective they are.

Our breakfast section, as a result, is oat-heavy. We have included some standard ways to eat oats as well as ideas that may surprise you, but we also know they will delight you when you try them.

My husband's successful, longstanding patients, some of whom have been on the program for nearly thirty years, *all* eat oats every day for breakfast! Evelyn calls them her favorite meal of the day; Anthony adds spinach and frozen vegetables to his; some cook them; some eat them as a cold cereal, but everyone eats them!

Be sure to add 1 to 2 tablespoons of ground flaxseeds or chia seeds to your oats every day to give them a boost of omega-3.

ESSY'S BREAKFAST BOWL

The genesis of everyone's breakfast in our family was my husband's breakfast. He has been eating it, unaltered, for at least forty years. He eats it every day, with almost no exceptions. And sometimes he has it after dinner, sort of as his dessert.

INGREDIENTS:

1 cup old-fashioned rolled oats

1 banana, sliced

1 tablespoon raisins

½ to 1 cup berries, such as blueberries, raspberries, and/or strawberries

1 to 2 tablespoons chia seeds or ground flaxseeds

¼ cup Ezekiel 4.9 or other nugget-type cereal for crunch (optional)

¼ cup unsweetened bite-size shredded wheat (optional)

1 cup unsweetened almond milk or oat milk

INSTRUCTIONS:

In a big bowl, combine the oats, banana, raisins, berries, chia seeds, and the cereals (if using). Top with nondairy milk, and go through the day with zip and joy!

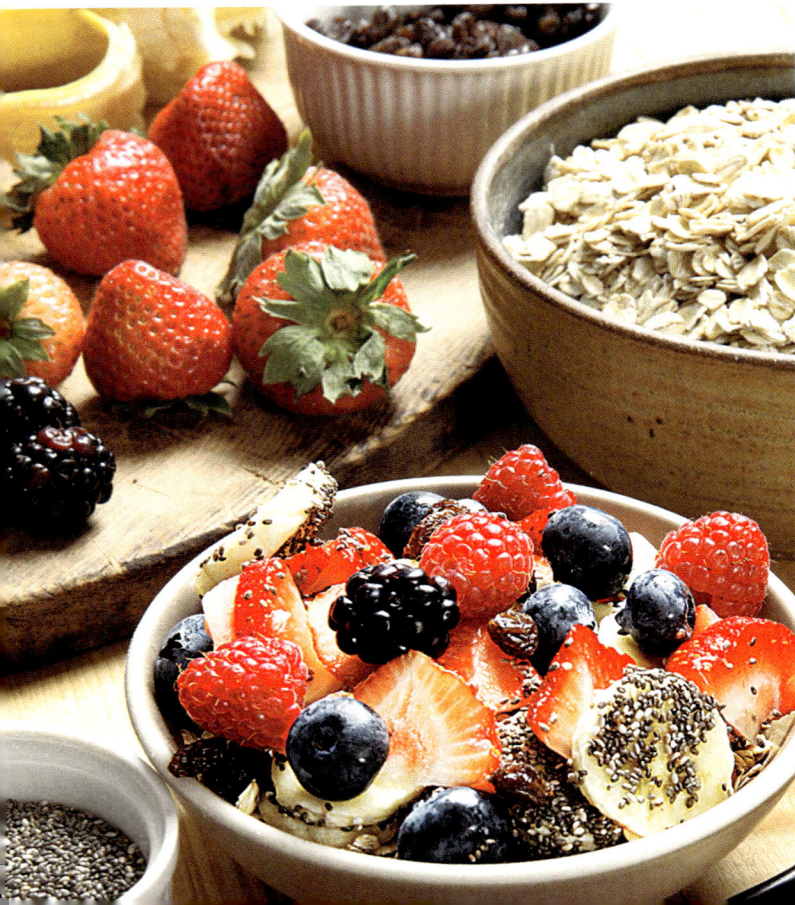

ANN'S OATS WITH GRAPES

I love oats this way! Be sure each bite has one sweet, wet grape in it! There is no liquid except the juice from the grapes. Jane says it's ridiculously dry. I love it! Other berries are good on this, too, as long as you still have a grape in every bite.

INGREDIENTS:

½ to ¾ cup old-fashioned rolled oats

8 to 12 grapes, halved

1 tablespoon chia seeds or ground
    flaxseeds

INSTRUCTIONS:

Put the oats in a bowl and top them with grapes and chia seeds, stir, and eat.

VARIATION:

For a delicious (more) wet cereal: Cut a grapefruit in half, remove the sections, and squeeze the juice over the oats. Add a sliced banana, sprinkle with chia seeds or ground flaxseeds, and top with any fresh or frozen berries.

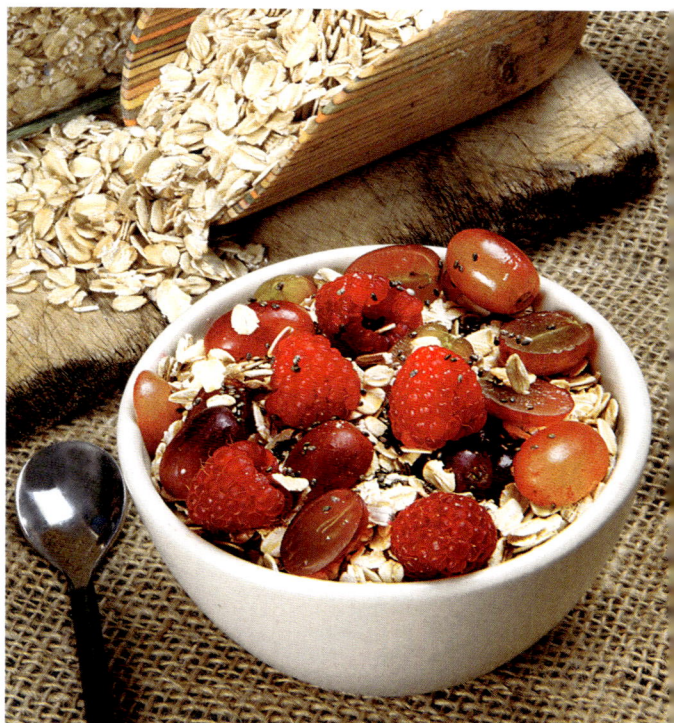

BANANA STEEL-CUT OATS

These steel-cut oats cooked in "banana milk" are good, and also easy. I have never liked oatmeal because I find it too mushy. Yet steel-cut oats don't get as mushy as old-fashioned oats, so when a woman told me she liked steel-cut oats cooked in mango "milk"—the blended liquid from a mango—I started experimenting. Make a triple batch of "banana milk"—I guarantee it is so delicious, you will want Banana Steel-Cut Oats for your next week of breakfasts! Make sure the banana is ripe! It is so sweet then. This breakfast tastes like banana bread. Try topping the oats with other types of berries, raisins, nutmeg, cinnamon, etc. These oats are also surprisingly sweet just alone.

INGREDIENTS:

1 large ripe banana

1 teaspoon pure vanilla extract

½ cup steel-cut oats

1 tablespoon ground flaxseeds or chia seeds

¼ cup frozen or fresh blueberries or other berries

INSTRUCTIONS:

In a food processor, combine the banana, vanilla, and 1 cup water. Process until smooth to create banana "milk."

Scrape the banana "milk" into a small saucepan, add the oats, and bring to a boil over high heat. Cover and reduce the heat to maintain a simmer. Simmer, stirring occasionally so the oats don't stick to the bottom, for 8 minutes. (If you like your oats less chewy, cook for a few minutes longer.) Remove from the heat.

The oats may look runny, but allow them to sit a few minutes to absorb some of the liquid. Serve the hot cereal in individual bowls, topped with the flaxseeds and blueberries.

VARIATION:

My niece Lili agrees with me about oatmeal being too mushy. She finds her steel-cut oats are perfect when they are made in a rice cooker! Her breakfast gets ready while she dresses for work—no stirring required. Give it a try, but follow the directions on the package for the water amount.

CINNAMON STICK OATMEAL

Our friend Norma from Mexico created this blend for us one morning. Norma was a national running champion for Mexico for a number of years and says that this oatmeal is a favorite meal for long-distance runners. But really, it's great for anyone who needs an extra energy boost for their day ahead. If you are having quinoa for dinner one night, make an extra cup and save it for the next morning to make this unbelievably delicious breakfast. It's nice with chopped apple or Norma's favorite way—with a chopped banana.

INGREDIENTS:

- 1 cinnamon stick
- 1 cup cooked quinoa
- 1 cup old-fashioned rolled oats, uncooked
- ¼ cup raisins
- Nondairy milk, for serving (optional)
- Sliced banana, apples, or berries, for serving (optional)

INSTRUCTIONS:

Put the cinnamon stick and 4 cups water into a saucepan and bring to a boil. Add the cooked quinoa and cook for 3 minutes. Add the oats, cover the pot, and reduce the heat to low. Cook for 15 minutes, until the oats are soft.

Remove from the heat, add the raisins, and let stand for 5 minutes.

Leave the cinnamon stick in for flavor, serve plain, *or* add some nondairy milk and sliced banana, apples, or berries.

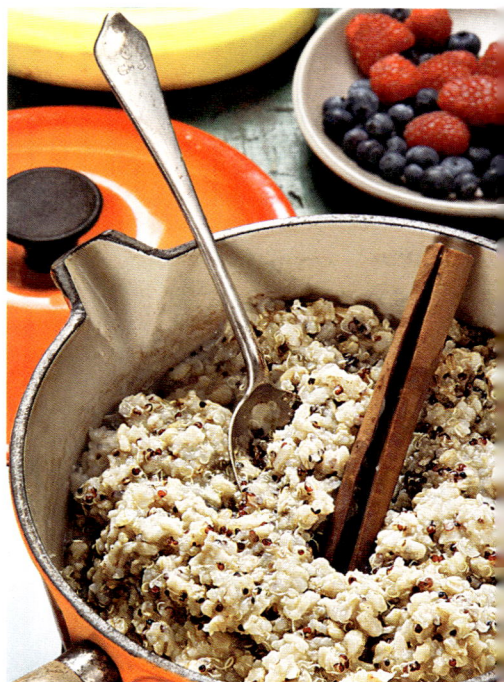

CHICKPEA OMELETS

When I first made these for my mom, she was skeptical. She doesn't like any dish that refers to eggs in any way (even if there's not an actual egg in sight). Yet after eating three of these "omelets," she decided they were wonderful and was amazed at the way the white pepper kicked in its unique flavor at the back of the throat.

INGREDIENTS:

1 cup chickpea flour

½ teaspoon onion powder

½ teaspoon garlic powder

¼ teaspoon white pepper

¼ teaspoon black pepper

⅓ cup nutritional yeast

½ teaspoon baking soda

1 cup water

3 green onions, chopped

4 ounces Sautéed Mushrooms (page 28; optional)

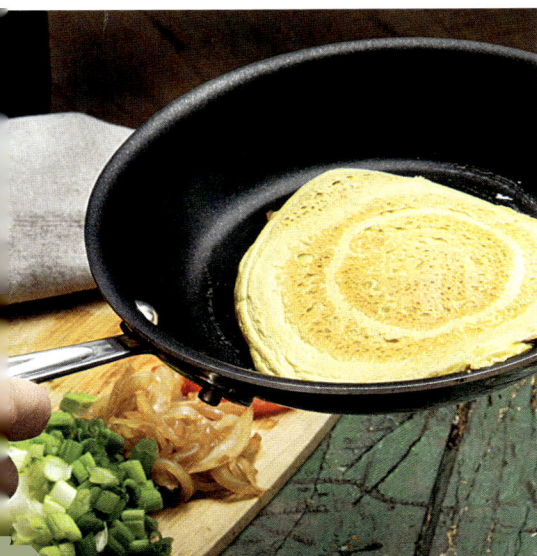

INSTRUCTIONS:

In a small bowl, combine the chickpea flour, onion powder, garlic powder, white pepper, black pepper, nutritional yeast, and baking soda. Add 1 cup water and stir until the batter is smooth.

Heat a frying pan over medium heat. Pour batter into the pan as if making pancakes. Sprinkle 1 to 2 tablespoons of the green onions and mushrooms into the batter for each omelet as it cooks. Flip the omelet like a pancake. When the underside is browned, flip the omelet again and cook the other side for a minute. Serve your amazing Chickpea Omelet with tomatoes, spinach, salsa, hot sauce, or whatever heart-safe, plant-perfect fixings you like.

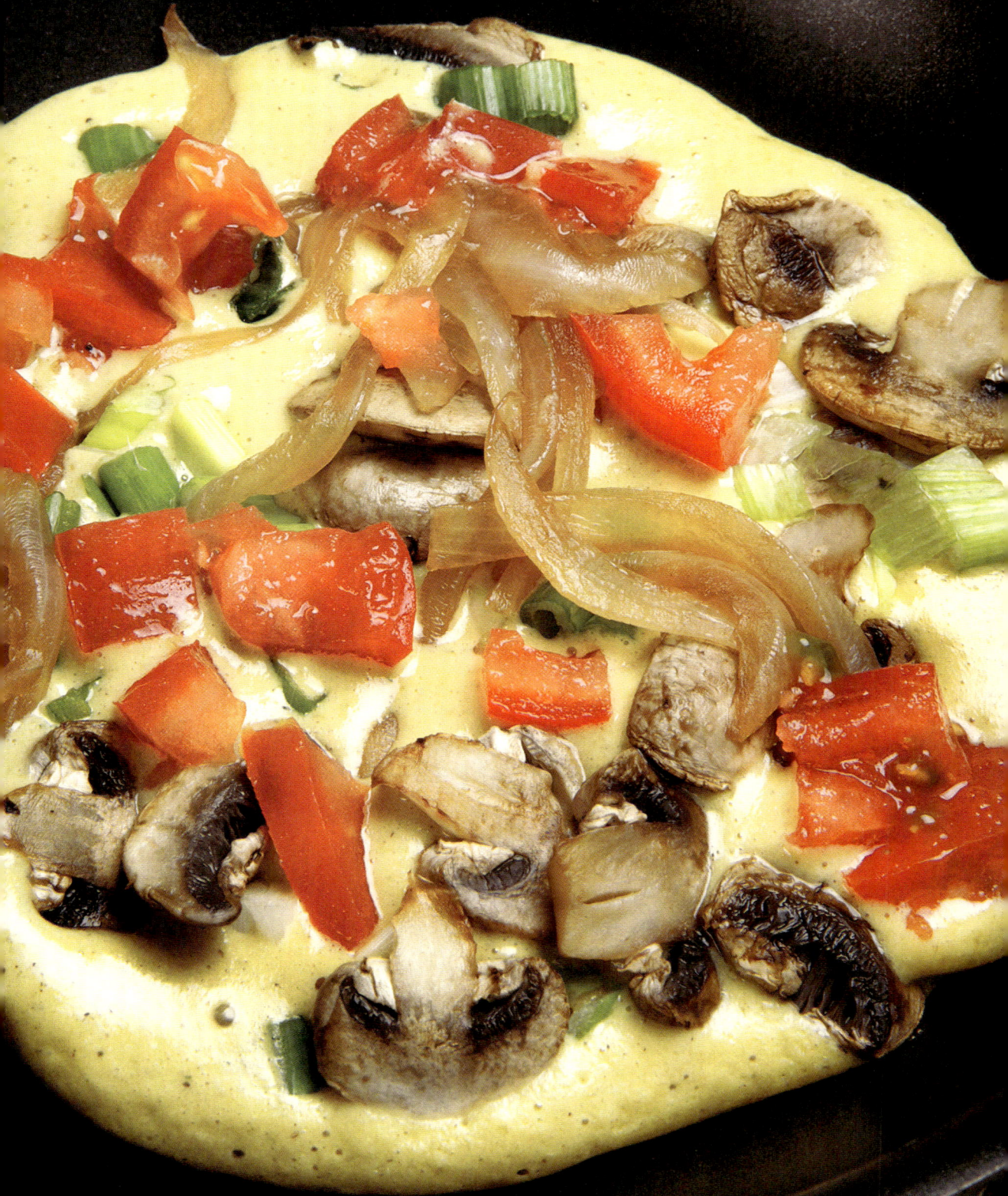

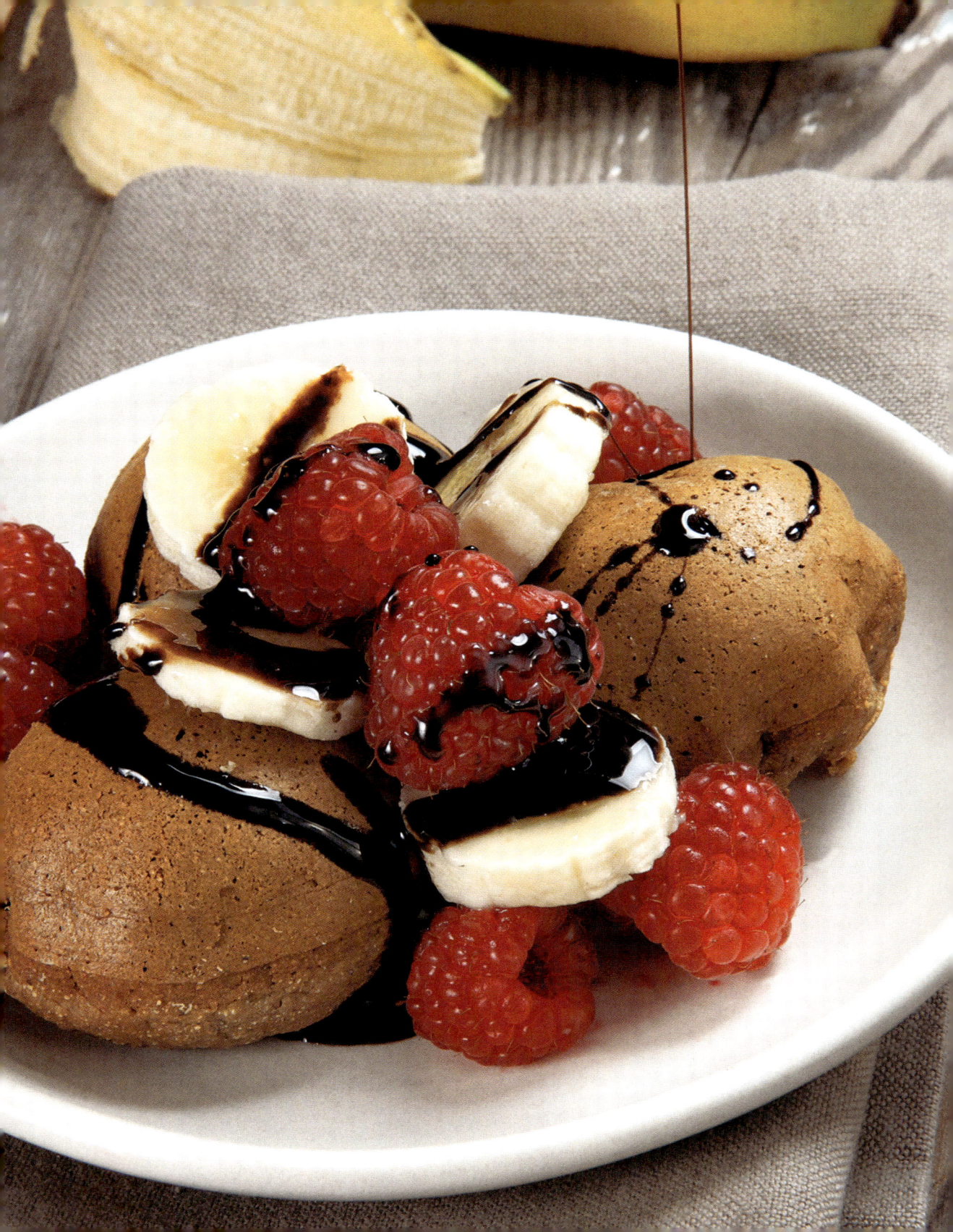

APPs: ADORABLE PANCAKE PUFFS

These looked so beautiful as I watched the woman in Williams-Sonoma make them, but the butter and eggs were a turnoff. Still, I bought the Ebelskiver Pancake Pan she was using. Ebelskiver is a traditional Danish pancake—sort of a cross between an American pancake and a popover! When I got home with my new ebelskiver pan, with its seven little wells, and started cooking, I expected to make little rocks, but I couldn't believe my results. My little Danish pancakes looked just as beautiful as the ones in the store, and they were way healthier. Below we have a savory recipe and a sweet recipe! Go get an ebelskiver pan—you'll need it for these adorable puffs!

SWEET VERSION

INGREDIENTS:

1 cup barley flour

½ teaspoon baking powder

2 tablespoons ground flaxseeds

1¼ cups plain unsweetened oat milk

3 tablespoons maple syrup, or to taste

½ teaspoon ground cinnamon

½ teaspoon vanilla extract

Chocolate balsamic vinegar, to taste

Berries, for serving

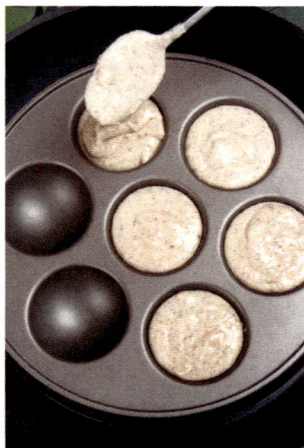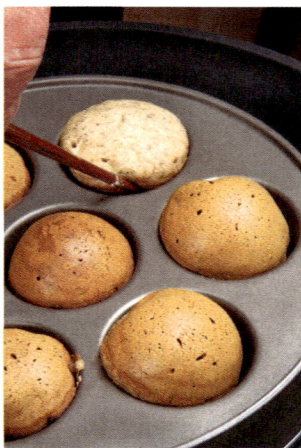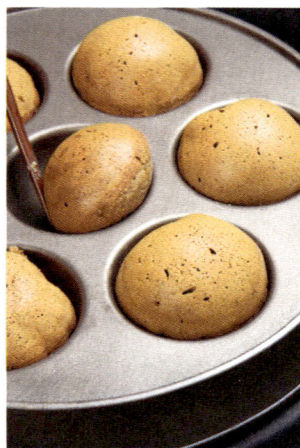

In a bowl, mix together the flour, baking powder, and flaxseeds. Add the oat milk, maple syrup, cinnamon, and vanilla, and stir to combine. Do not over-mix.

Heat the *ebelskiver* pan over medium heat. Place 1 tablespoon of the batter in each well. Cook until the bottoms are golden brown, about 5 minutes. Use a wooden skewer to tip the pancakes over, and cook for 3 to 5 minutes on the other side, until golden brown.

Eat each bite with a berry or two and a drizzle of chocolate balsamic vinegar!

SAVORY VERSION

2 cups uncooked kale, Swiss chard, or other greens, chopped into very small pieces

1 tablespoon balsamic vinegar

1 cup barley flour or any whole-grain flour

½ teaspoon baking powder

2 tablespoons ground flaxseeds

1 cup plain unsweetened almond milk or oat milk

1 cup frozen corn, thawed

1 jalapeño, seeded and diced

4 green onions, white and green parts chopped

¼ cup salsa (optional)

Place the kale in a saucepan and add enough water to cover. Bring the water to a boil, cover, and cook for 4 to 5 minutes, until the kale is soft. Drain in a colander, squeeze out the excess water, and transfer to a bowl. If there are still long pieces of kale, chop them into smaller pieces with kitchen shears. Mix in the balsamic vinegar.

In a bowl, combine the flour, baking powder, and flaxseeds. Add the almond milk, corn, jalapeños, and green onions.

Heat the *ebelskiver* pan over medium-low heat. Add 1 tablespoon of the batter to each well. Plop a layer of the cooked greens on the uncooked batter in the wells, then top each well with another tablespoon of batter.

Cook until the bottoms are golden brown, about 5 minutes. Be patient and wait to turn until batter has browned. Use a wooden skewer to tip the pancakes over, and cook for 3 to 5 minutes on the other side, until golden brown.

Dip each bite into a little salsa, if you like. So good!

BREAKFAST HASH

We serve this at Engine 2 Retreats and Immersions for breakfast—mostly because it gives us a chance to teach about the taste and satiating powers of yummy fresh salsas!

INGREDIENTS:

1 large onion, diced

1 red bell pepper, diced

1 green bell pepper, diced

2 large Yukon Gold potatoes, cooked, cooled, and cut into ½-inch cubes

1 (16-ounce) can black beans, drained and rinsed

½ teaspoon garlic powder, or to taste

¼ teaspoon freshly ground black pepper

Mango-Lime Salsa (page 120), Pico de Gallo (page 119), or another salsa of your choice, for serving

Hot sauce, ketchup, or Enchilada Sauce (page 114), for serving (optional)

INSTRUCTIONS:

Heat a frying pan over high heat. Add the onions and cook, stirring continuously, until the onions are translucent and have browned a bit. Add a few drops of water if the pan gets dry.

Reduce the heat to medium and add the red and green bell peppers and the potato cubes. Cook until the potato cubes are browned and the peppers are cooked through.

Add the black beans and continue to cook, stirring. Season with garlic powder and black pepper to taste.

Serve warm, with a huge variety of fresh salsas and hot sauce, ketchup, or enchilada sauce.

ALL-OAT WAFFLES

For breakfast there are three things I want to eat every day: oats, chia seeds or ground flaxseeds, and a banana. That is exactly what these waffles allow me to do! I have made many versions of these waffles, starting one day when I simply poured my breakfast oats into the waffle iron! Eat them with a berry in every waffle hole, covered with applesauce, Raspberry Sauce (page 113), or the tiniest bit of maple syrup. Or enjoy them just plain. Helpful hint: A good nonstick waffle iron and a wooden chopstick are key!

INGREDIENTS:

1 very ripe small to medium banana

1 cup old-fashioned oats

½ cup water or nondairy milk

2 tablespoons ground flaxseeds or chia seeds

1 teaspoon vanilla extract

Zest of ½ orange, or more if you prefer, or ½ to 1 teaspoon orange extract

INSTRUCTIONS:

Preheat a waffle iron.

Place the banana in a food processor and process until smooth.

Add the oats, water, flaxseeds, vanilla, and orange zest to the food processor with the banana and blend until smooth and only flecks of oats are visible. The batter will be thick.

All waffle irons are different, so follow the directions for yours, or try ⅓ cup batter for each 4-inch square waffle section. Close the lid, set a timer for 8 minutes, and don't peek or attempt to remove the waffles before the 8 minutes are up. If the iron is hard to open after 8 minutes, cook the waffles a little longer. If the waffles stick, use a chopstick to remove them. They are still good even if they come out in little pieces!

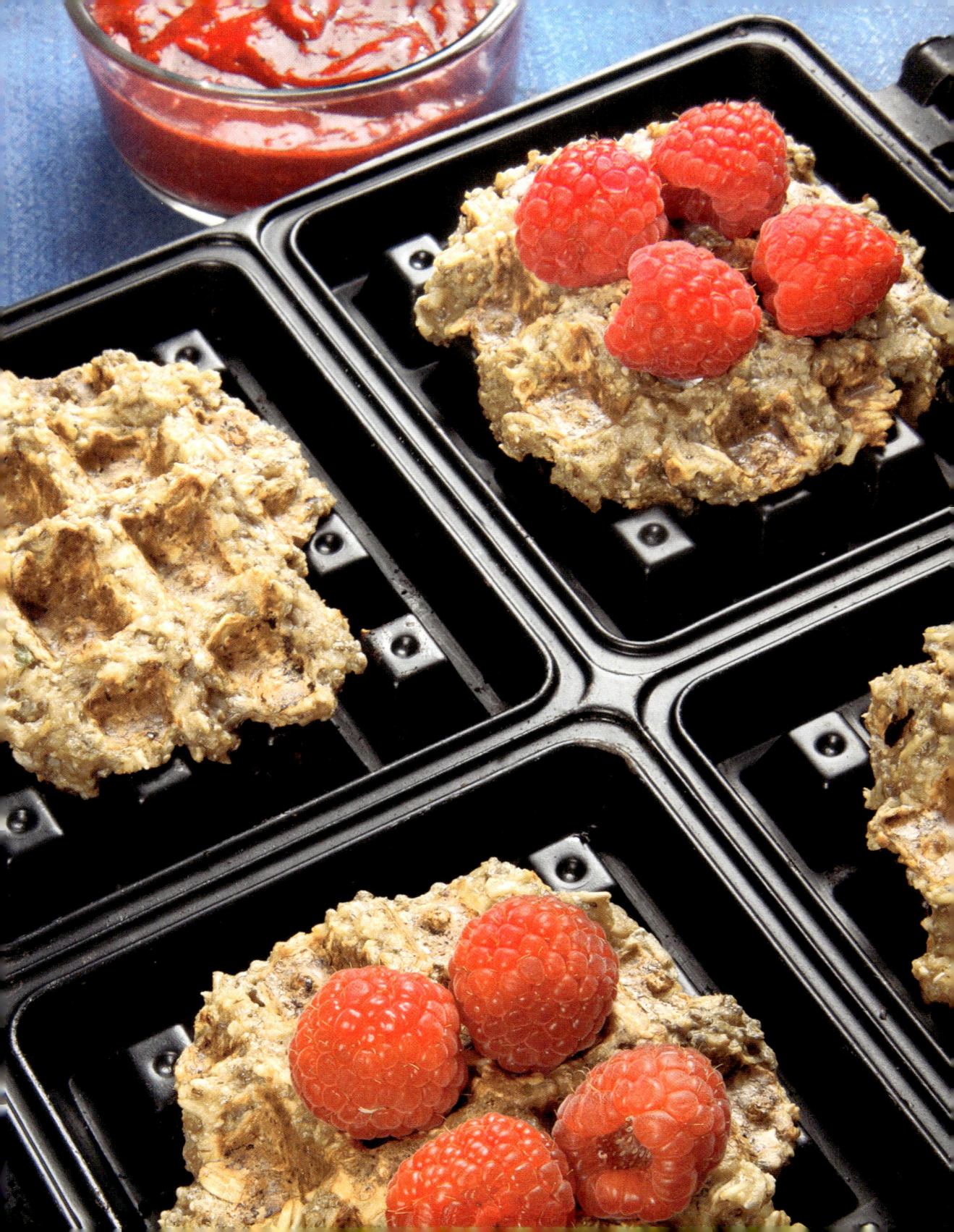

SAVORY SMOKY OATS

I don't like hot oatmeal, but this is different! This recipe evolved from a post on Debbie Kastner's Happy Healthy Long Life *blog featuring her savory oats breakfast creation, which she calls "A Mega-Nitric Oxide Antioxidant Boosting Breakfast for Champions." We fired it up here with liquid smoke. If it seems too runny after ten minutes, you will find it is just right when it is filled with greens! The problem with this is eating just one serving! It also works at any meal—Jane likes it for dinner.*

INGREDIENTS:

- ½ cup steel-cut oats
- ½ cup dried shiitake mushrooms, sliced (about ½ ounce), or ½ cup fresh shiitakes
- 3 tablespoons nutritional yeast
- ¼ teaspoon ground turmeric
- 7 ounces diced or crushed no-salt-added tomatoes
- ¼ teaspoon liquid smoke
- ½ teaspoon garlic powder
- ½ teaspoon onion powder
- 1 cup spinach
- Freshly ground black pepper
- Hot sauce of choice, such as sriracha or Cholula (optional)

INSTRUCTIONS:

In a saucepan, combine the oats, mushrooms, nutritional yeast, turmeric, tomatoes, liquid smoke, garlic powder, onion powder, and 1½ cups water. Bring the mixture to a boil, watching carefully and stirring to prevent scorching. When the mixture just comes to a boil, reduce the heat to maintain a simmer and cook, stirring occasionally, for 10 minutes, until the water has been absorbed and the oats are creamy.

Add the spinach and black pepper to taste, and stir until the spinach is mixed in (or you can also add spinach to each individual bowl). Eat as-is or with a dab of hot sauce. Oh my, it is good!

You can make this recipe using 1 cup chopped kale or Swiss chard. You'll just need to cook these greens longer. You can either cook them in advance and add them to your bowl or add the greens to the pan with the other ingredients after the oat mixture has been cooking for 5 minutes.

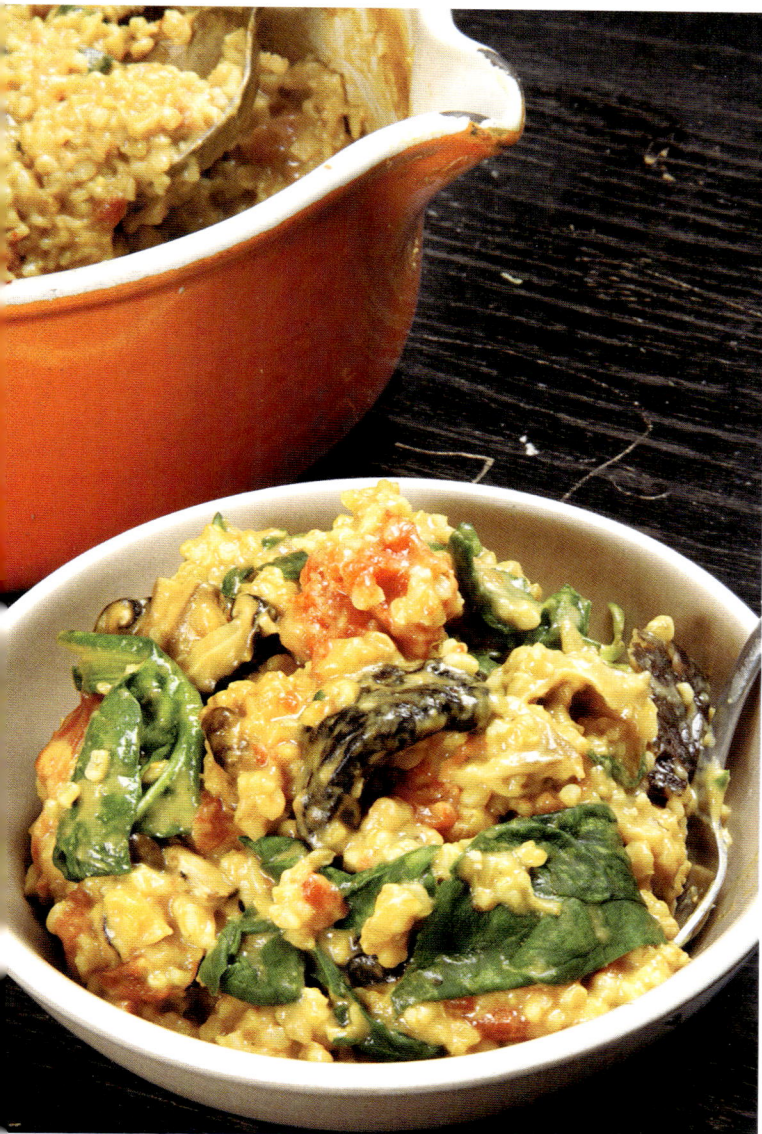

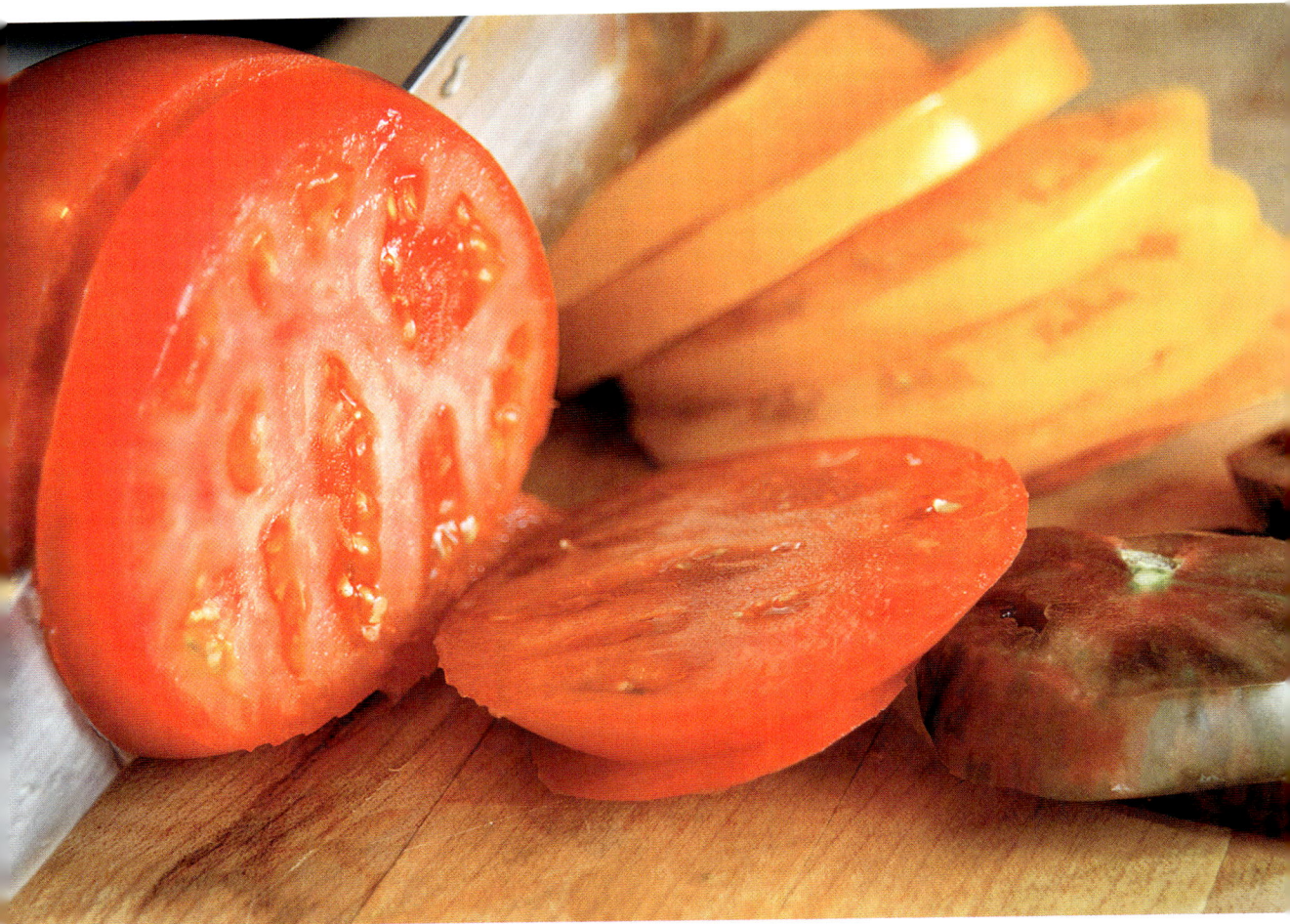

LUNCHES

Along with soup for lunch, sandwiches are favorites for us, especially vegetable-filled open-faced sandwiches. One of our favorites is our kale sandwich. Oh, we love that! Another is the tomato-basil one we have *every day* from the beginning of delicious summer tomatoes until the first frost. Warm and hearty vegetable-stuffed paninis are another favorite, as are our wraps filled with hummus and vegetables and baked in the oven until crispy. Truly, anything between good whole-grain bread with lots of hummus and even more vegetables is delicious!

All these sandwiches are such fun, and there are so many yummy variations. We feel creative and magical when we try out different sandwich combinations. Lunch becomes a form of "wich-craft"!

CUCUMBER AND KALE OPEN-FACED SANDWICH

The layer of kale and mustard together in this sandwich is delicious, particularly when you use a great mustard. We love True Natural Taste Sweet and Spicy Creamy White Mustard, available at truenaturaltaste.com.

INGREDIENTS:

2 slices whole-grain bread, toasted

2 to 3 tablespoons Our Hummus (page 102) or hummus prepared without oil or tahini

1 green onion, chopped

¼ cup fresh cilantro, chopped

2 medium kale leaves, chopped into bite-size pieces (about the size of cilantro leaves)

½ small cucumber

Mustard of choice

Lemon pepper (Mrs. Dash and Frontier brands have no salt)

INSTRUCTIONS:

Spread the toasted bread generously with hummus. Sprinkle the green onion, cilantro, and kale evenly over the hummus.

Slice the cucumber into 8 rounds and spread each round with a thin layer of mustard.

Place the cucumber rounds, mustard-side down, on top of the cilantro-kale layer, and press down, if necessary, so they stay in place.

Sprinkle the open-faced sandwich generously with lemon pepper, cut in half or quarters, if desired, and serve.

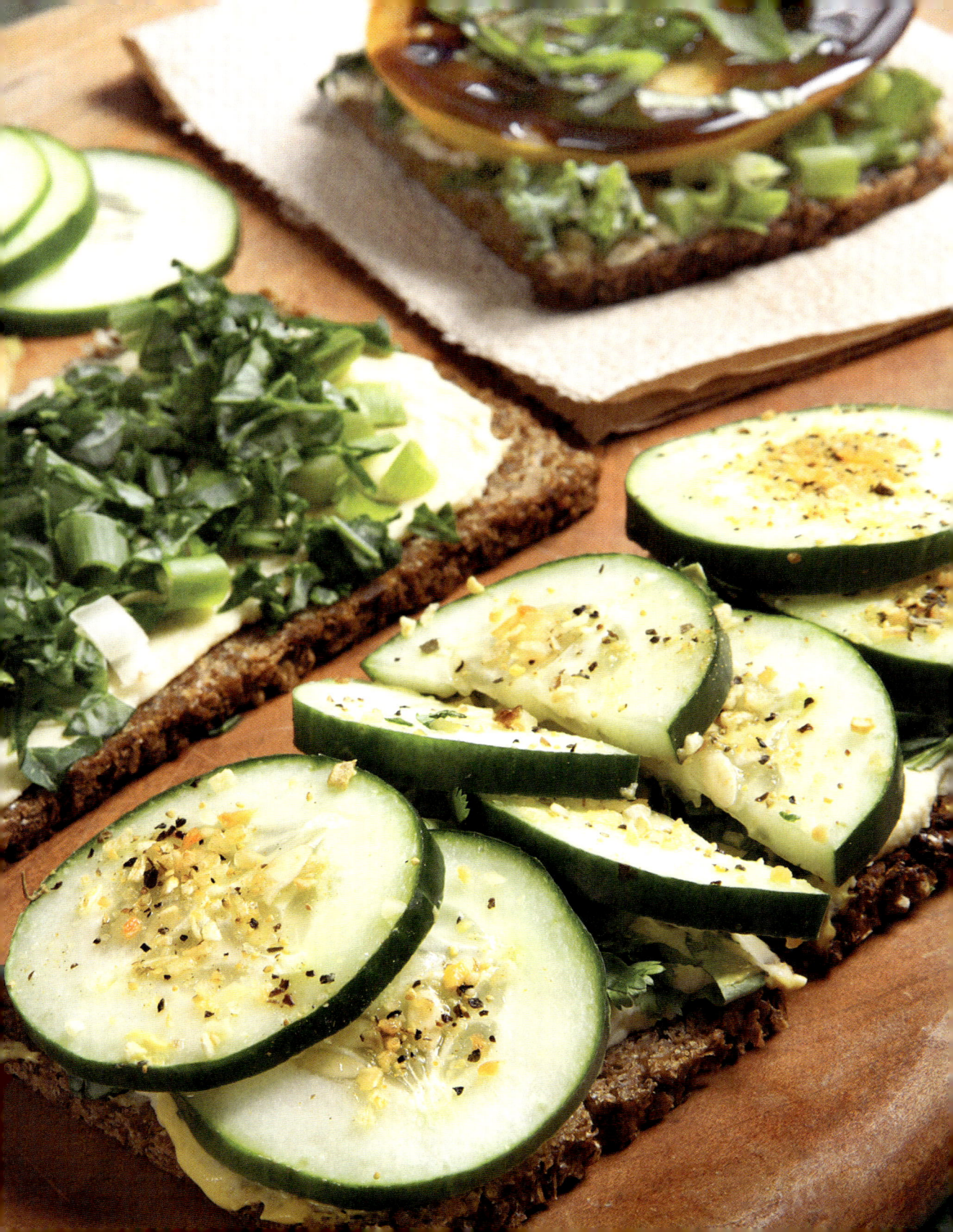

KALE BRUSCHETTA

We adore this as an appetizer, and so does everyone else. It is always the first empty platter at our holiday party. No one knows it is plant-based; they just know it is so yummy. This is a no-nuts, "enlightened" version of the Kale Bruschetta recipe from My Beef with Meat.

INGREDIENTS:

1 bunch Cooked Kale (page 23)

1 loaf fresh 100 percent whole-grain bread, sliced (find a great rustic whole-grain loaf from a healthy bakery)

½ cup Cannellini Bean Sauce (page 110)

1 cup grape tomatoes, halved

Balsamic glaze, preferably Isola Classic Cream of Balsamic

INSTRUCTIONS:

Squeeze any extra liquid out of the kale with your hands. You don't want soggy bread.

Toast as many pieces of bread as desired and place on a handsome serving platter.

Spread the cannellini sauce on the toasted bread.

Layer the kale over the cannellini sauce. Scatter the grape tomatoes over the kale. Drizzle generously with the balsamic glaze, and grab one for yourself before they all disappear.

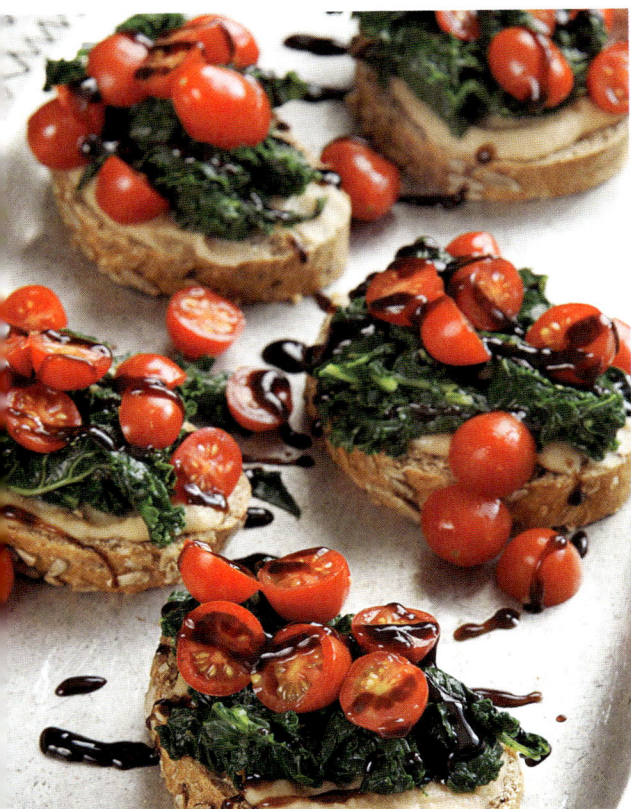

THICK HEIRLOOM TOMATO OPEN-FACED SANDWICH

These are so good, we eat them every day *from the time the first heirloom tomato ripens in our garden until the sad end of these beauties. If you don't have heirloom tomatoes (Brandywine are our favorite), any large summer tomato works. Mestemacher or Feldkamp bread (rectangular, dense, thinly sliced, dark rye) is available in health food stores; alternatively, use a dark, coarse rye or whole-grain bread of your choice.*

INGREDIENTS:

- 2 pieces Mestemacher or Feldkamp bread, or 4 slices whole-grain bread of choice
- 4 to 6 tablespoons Our Hummus (page 102) or hummus prepared without oil or tahini
- 2 green onions, chopped
- 2 medium kale leaves, chopped to the size of the green onions
- 8 large basil leaves, chopped (about ¼ cup)
- 1 large heirloom or regular tomato, cut into 4 thick slices
- 3 to 4 tablespoons balsamic vinegar

INSTRUCTIONS:

Toast, or better yet double or triple toast, the bread until it holds together well.

Spread the toasted bread with lots of hummus and top with the green onions, kale, and basil.

Cut the bread in half at this point (because it is so long), and then place a tomato slice on each piece.

Sprinkle the tomato with balsamic vinegar and spread it around a bit with a knife or your finger. Enjoy summer's ambrosia!

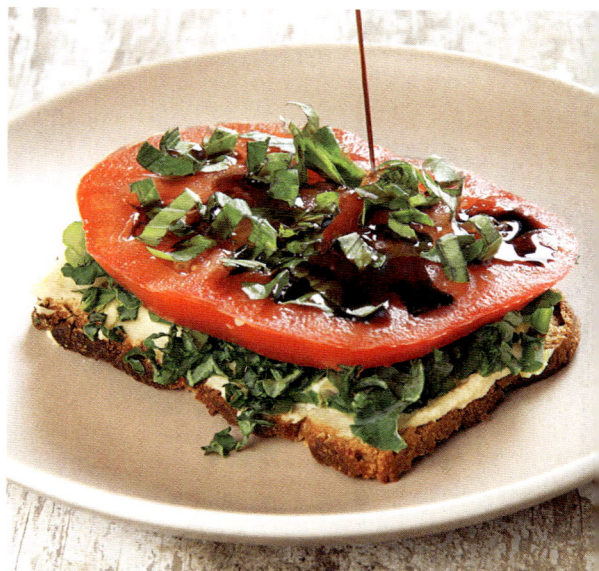

THE ULTIMATE: LEMON AND KALE OPEN-FACED SANDWICH

When we came up with this recipe, we had been traveling and longed for greens, and when we got home only kale was in the refrigerator. Lucky for us that day! This sandwich is stunningly delicious and tastes as good as it is healthy. Any leafy green—kale, Swiss chard, spinach—will work. The lemon adds an almost sweet taste. Be generous with it—lots of lemon juice makes this sandwich so good!

INGREDIENTS:

2 slices Mestemacher or Feldkamp bread, or 4 slices whole-grain bread of choice

1 bunch Cooked Kale (page 23) or greens of choice

4 to 6 tablespoons Our Hummus (page 102) or hummus prepared without oil or tahini

4 green onions, sliced

½ bunch cilantro or parsley, chopped

2 lemons

1 large tomato, cut into 4 thick slices (optional)

Lemon pepper (Mrs. Dash and Frontier brands have no salt)

INSTRUCTIONS:

Toast, or better yet double or triple toast, the bread until it holds together well.

Squeeze any extra liquid out of the kale with your hands and set it aside in a colander. You don't want soggy bread.

Spread the toasted bread with lots of hummus and top evenly with the green onions and a pile of cilantro. Cut each piece of bread in half.

Cut one of the lemons in half with a very sharp knife, then slice into about 8 very skinny lemon slices, cutting from the centers of each half outward. (This guarantees less rind and pith per bite.) Cut each round into quarters—this ensures that when you take a bite, the whole lemon slice won't come off the sandwich all at once. Scatter the thin lemon slices all over each open-faced sandwich.

Zest and juice the remaining lemon. Sprinkle the kale in the colander with lemon zest and juice and toss. Arrange a big handful of lemony kale on top of each piece of bread and then sprinkle with lemon pepper.

Serve—or top with a tomato slice and lemon pepper. Health in each bite—a bit of a messy one, at that!

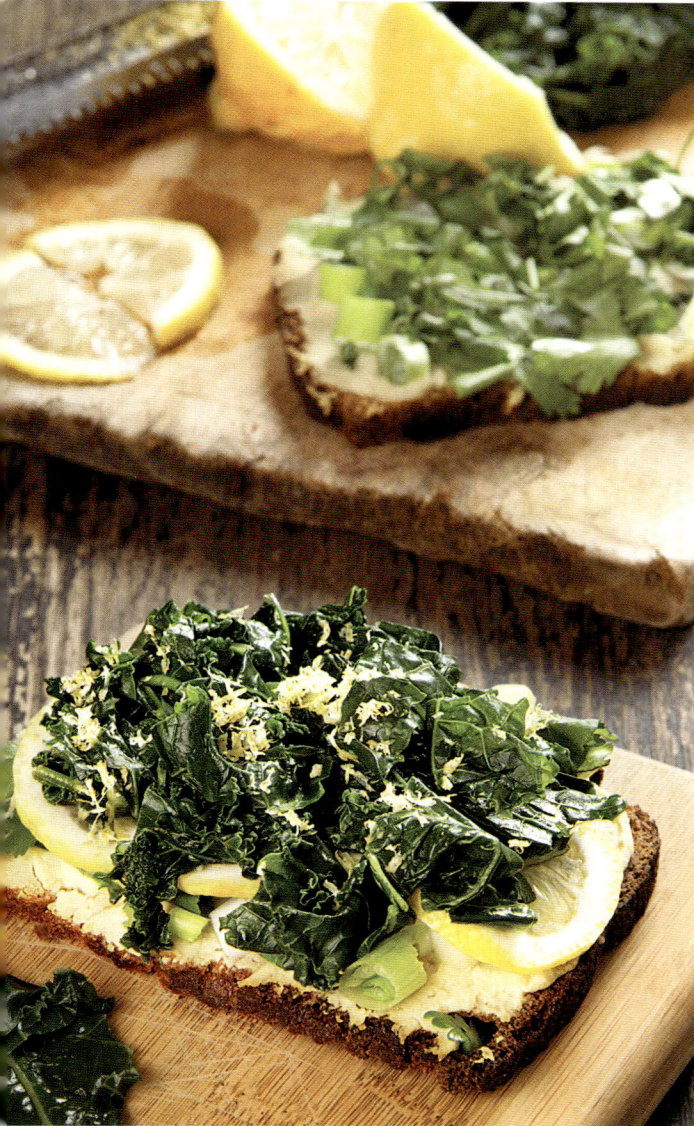

KALE AND SAUERKRAUT SANDWICH

We were never particularly big sauerkraut enthusiasts, but after we discovered this sandwich, that was no longer true. I learned about this extraordinary flavor combination from a friend and had to try it. Fortunately, we had a jar of sauerkraut in the refrigerator left over from when our son Zeb, who likes it, was visiting. I used the Engine 2 Jalapeño Cilantro Hummus and a horseradish mustard the first time I made this, and I was blown away by the taste. Sauerkraut is a high-sodium food, so choose a lower-sodium brand, such as Eden Organic or Bubbies, and then rinse and drain the sauerkraut before using it. If you are using plain hummus, add a big sprinkle of lemon pepper on top.

INGREDIENTS:

4 slices whole-grain bread

4 tablespoons Our Hummus (page 102) or hummus prepared with no tahini or oil (Engine 2 Jalapeño Cilantro is recommended)

3 to 4 tablespoons prepared horseradish mustard or other mustard of your choice

1 bunch Cooked Kale (page 23) or greens of choice

½ cup prepared sauerkraut, rinsed and drained

8 cherry tomatoes, halved, or 1 small tomatoes, sliced

INSTRUCTIONS:

Preheat a panini press.

Lay the slices of bread in pairs. Spread one slice of each pairing with the hummus and the other slice with the mustard.

Squeeze any extra liquid out of the kale with your hands. Do the same with the sauerkraut. You don't want soggy bread.

Spread a layer of kale on top of the hummus, then spread a layer of sauerkraut on top of the kale, and tomatoes on top of the sauerkraut. Place the mustard-covered bread on top, mustard-side down.

Heat the sandwiches in the panini press until brown and warmed through. Cut on an angle and serve. You'll be surprised by the taste combination!

DAGWOOD SANDWICH

A friend called the other day saying she could go plant-based no problem, as long as she could have the darn good sandwich she had just eaten every day of the week! I asked her what was in this "darn good" sandwich. Well, it was amazing—so amazing we have named it the Dagwood Sandwich—in honor of the stunningly enormous sandwiches made by Dagwood in the long-running Blondie *cartoon.*

INGREDIENTS:

8 slices Ezekiel Bread or other whole-grain bread made with no oil

8 ounces Our Hummus (page 102) or hummus prepared with no tahini or oil

8 green-leaf lettuce or spinach leaves, or more as desired

1 cucumber, sliced

1 cup Sautéed Mushrooms (page 28; try variation 2 made with Bone Suckin' Sauce—our favorite barbecue sauce!)

1 cup Roasted Red Peppers (page 24)

4 rounds Grilled Pineapple (page 29)

½ cup Caramelized Onions (page 27)

2 large tomatoes, sliced

12 dill pickle slices (optional)

INSTRUCTIONS:

Lay the slices of bread in pairs. Spread hummus on each slice of bread. Place a lettuce leaf on one slice of each pair. Add a few slices of cucumber on top of the lettuce. Add Sautéed Mushrooms and a few Roasted Red Peppers on top of the cucumber.

Place a round of Grilled Pineapple and a layer of Caramelized Onions on top of the peppers.

Add a large slice of tomato on top of the Caramelized Onions.

Add a few pickles, if you wish.

Top with the hummus-coated piece of bread, hummus-side down. Insert a long toothpick (it may have to be a shish-kebab skewer!) and serve.

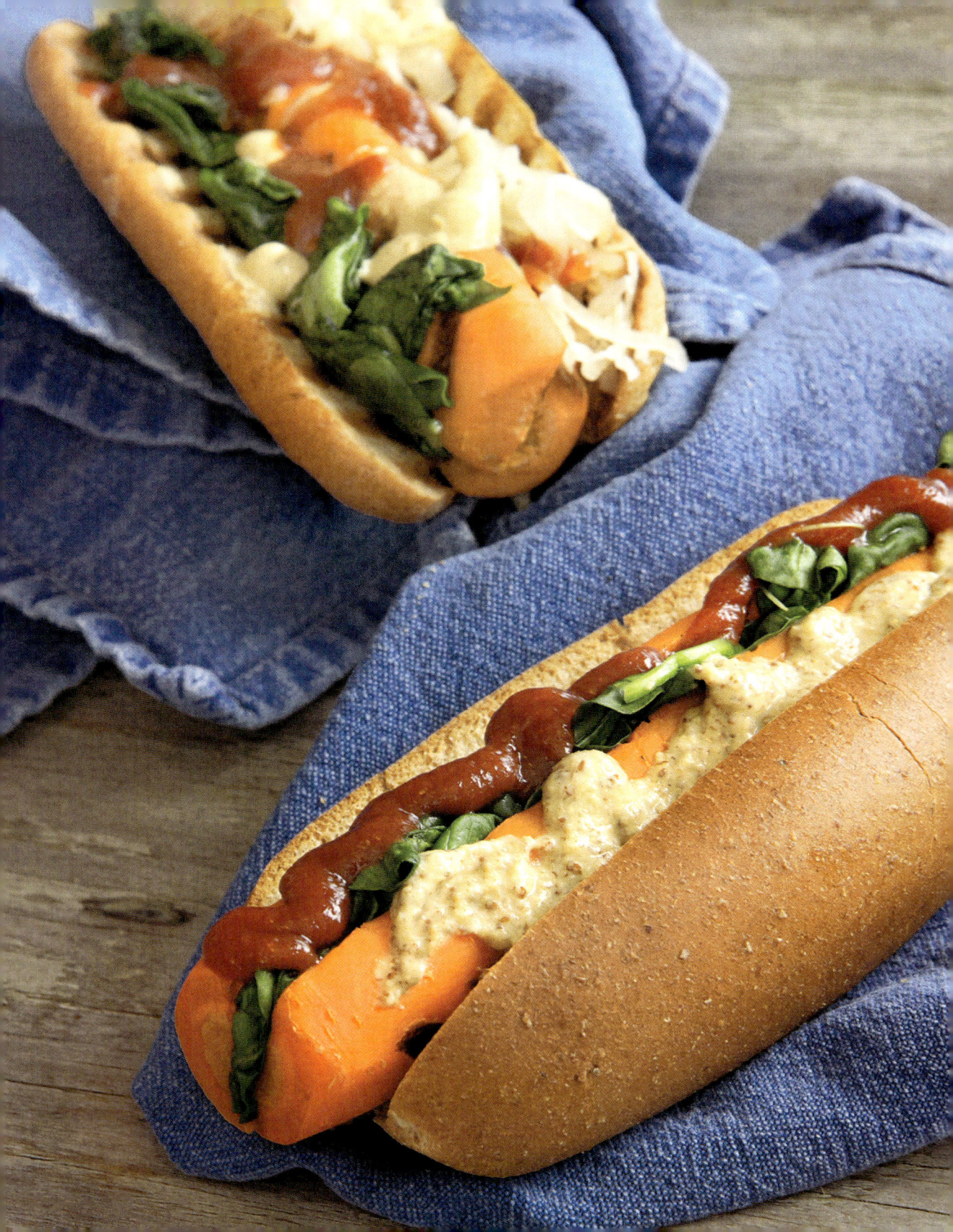

CARROT DOGS

We used to recommend Smart Dogs for an occasional cookout treat, even though they are highly processed. But now, Smart Dogs have been reformulated to be "grillable," meaning the company that makes them has added oil (it's even listed as the second ingredient in the ingredients list). So, Smart Dogs are no longer an option. But their replacement may surprise you: Carrot Dogs! You can make these Carrot Dogs in a panini press, or grill them up at a summer block party!

INGREDIENTS:

2 long, straight carrots (hot dog length and size, but not too long or too thick)

1 teaspoon liquid smoke

2 whole wheat hot-dog buns, or 2 slices whole-grain bread
   (Ezekiel Low-Sodium brand is our favorite)

Fixings:

- Spinach—cooked and drained, or fresh
- Ketchup
- Mustard
- Sauerkraut
- Caramelized Onions (page 27)

INSTRUCTIONS:

Preheat a panini press, or heat an outdoor grill.

Bring a large pot of water to a boil. Add the carrots and boil for 10 to 15 minutes, or until they are hot dog–like soft. Stick a knife or fork in one to be sure.

Drain the carrots, cut them in half lengthwise, and rub liquid smoke on all sides with a knife or your finger.

Place the carrots flat in the panini press or on the grill, and grill until lightly browned, just a few minutes. If space allows, put the bread or bun, opened, alongside the carrot to toast it a little.

Place the carrot in the bun and top with the spinach, ketchup, and mustard. Finally, add some sauerkraut and Caramelized Onions.

Can you believe it!? The world's healthiest Carrot Dog!

LETTUCE WRAPS WITH CREAMY MARINATED VEGETABLES

The filling in these glorious lettuce wraps has the most fabulous combination of tastes. Don't be afraid to use the jalapeño and garlic. They don't jump out too strongly—they just add to the wonderful flavor. Use white balsamic vinegar if you want to keep the color brighter. The filling is delicious in lettuce wraps, in pitas, or in any sandwiches. It's really good by the spoonful, too!

INGREDIENTS:

2 large carrots, thinly sliced into rounds or matchsticks

1 red bell pepper, seeded and chopped

½ cucumber, quartered, seeded, and chopped

4 green onions, chopped

½ cup fresh cilantro, chopped

1 small jalapeño, seeded and chopped (you can start with just half, but be bold!)

1 clove garlic, chopped

4 tablespoons balsamic vinegar or vinegar of choice

8 ounces Our Hummus (page 102) or hummus prepared with no tahini or oil

1 to 2 heads Bibb or butter lettuce (enough to find 12 whole leaves)

INSTRUCTIONS:

In a bowl, toss together the carrots, bell pepper, cucumber, green onions, cilantro, jalapeño, and garlic. Add the vinegar, stir, and then add the hummus. Stir again, cover, and refrigerate until ready to use.

To make the lettuce wraps, fill the center of a lettuce leaf with about ¼ cup of the dressed vegetables. Arrange the filled leaves on a platter. To eat, fold the sides together into a little wrap.

TIP:

To use this filling in sandwiches, generously cover both sides of pita or bread with a little more hummus, add a small handful of spinach and a pile of vegetables, and you have a drippy feast of wonderful tastes ahead of you.

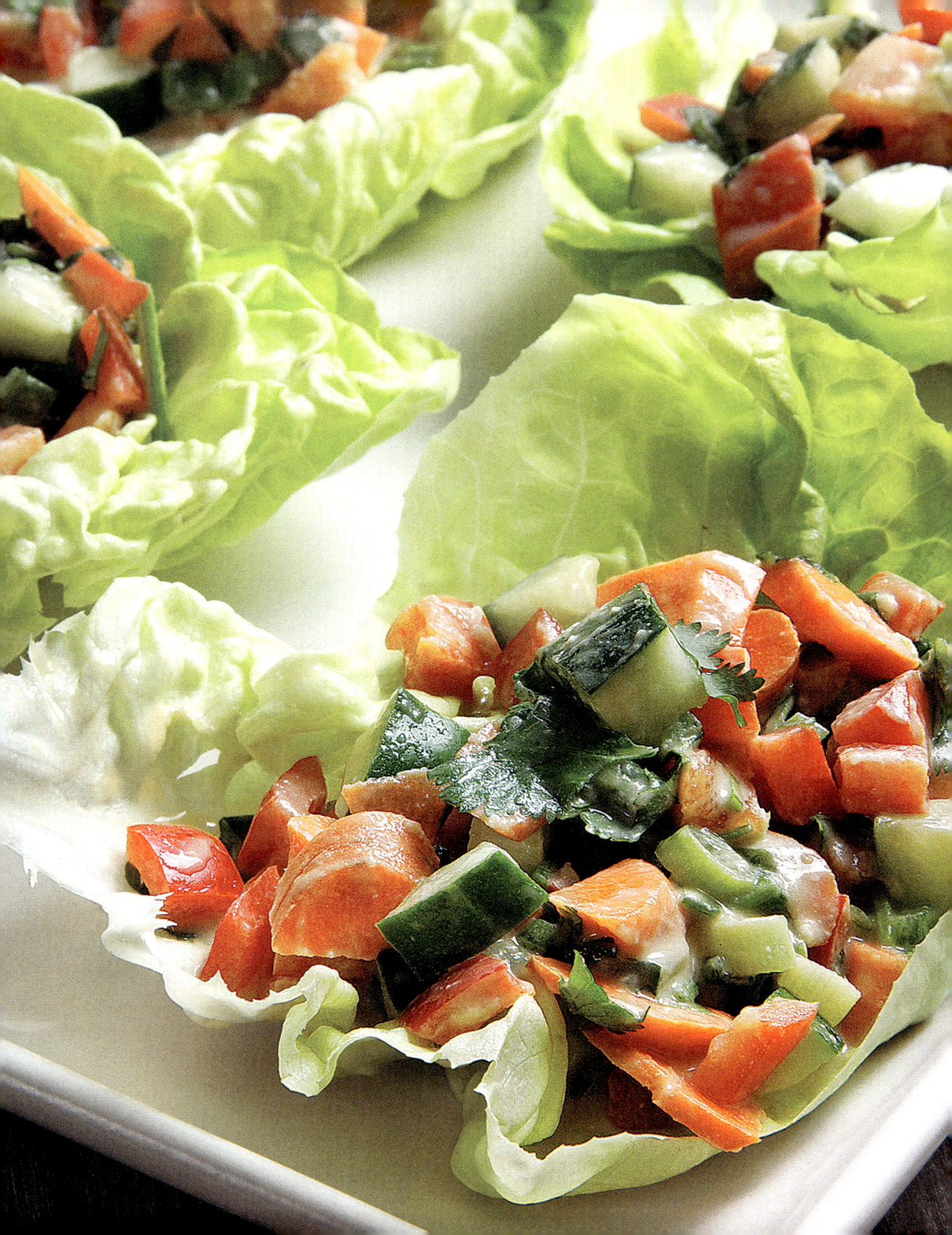

LOVELY COLLARD SUSHI

These are stunningly beautiful and delicious. They are such fun to make—it doesn't feel like work. Substitute cooked asparagus or green beans, long carrots, bok choy strips, cooked greens, anything for the filling. Fresh basil gives them a strong bite, too. Really, anything is good in them. They make perfect sushi-like hors d'oeuvres, or eat them for lunch instead of a sandwich. Collards are pretty tough and don't easily break apart when cooked. Their flexibility makes them a perfect wrap.

INGREDIENTS:

1 bunch collards

8 tablespoons Our Hummus (page 102) or hummus prepared with no tahini or oil

2 green onions, chopped

½ cup fresh cilantro, chopped

¼ cup shredded carrots

¼ red bell pepper, seeded and cut into thin strips

¼ small cucumber, peeled, if desired, and cut into thin strips

½ mango, pitted, peeled, and cut into thin strips

Zest and juice of 2 lemons

INSTRUCTIONS:

Fill a frying pan with about 2 inches of water and bring to a boil.

Choose four of the nicest-looking collard leaves. Lay them flat, cut off the thick stem at the point where the leaf begins, then carefully stack the leaves on top of one another in the boiling water. Cover and cook for about 30 seconds.

Drain the collards and lay them flat on a dry cutting board or counter with the thick part of the spine facing up. The leaves need to be dry. If they are still wet, pat them dry with a paper towel.

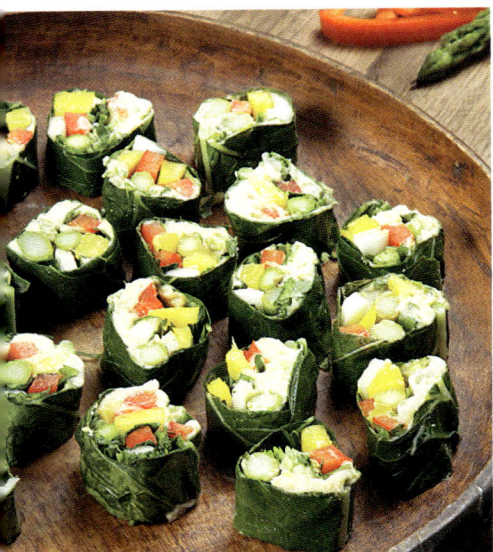

Down the center spine of each collard leaf, spread about 2 tablespoons of the hummus, and then sprinkle generously with green onions, cilantro, and shredded carrots. Place bell pepper, cucumber, and mango strips on top.

Sprinkle with lemon zest and a generous amount of lemon juice. Lemon makes it good!

Starting with the side nearest to you, gently roll the leaf and filling into a sausage shape, tucking the edges in as you roll.

With a sharp knife, cut the roll into as many *small* pieces as possible. You should be able to get 6 or more pieces, but it will depend on the size of the collard leaf. The roller always gets to eat the end pieces!

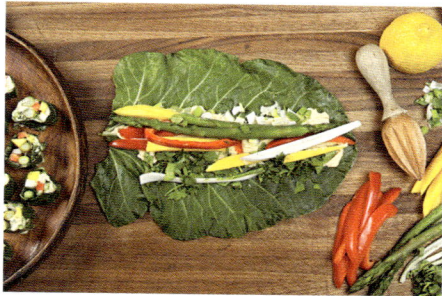

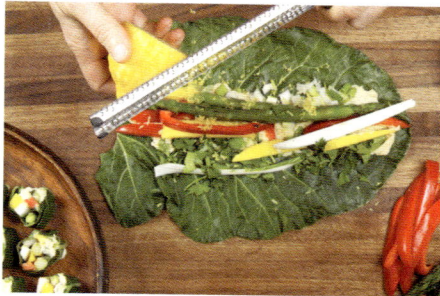

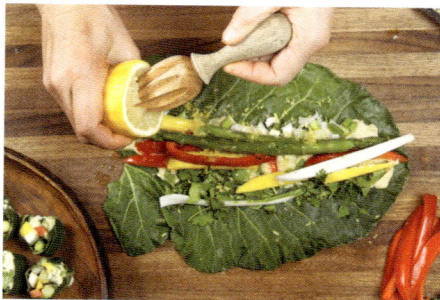

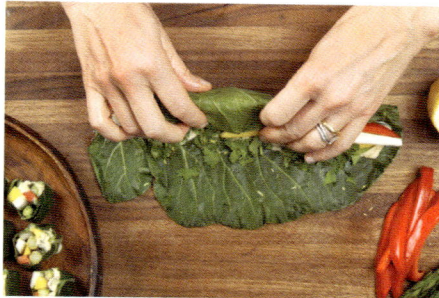

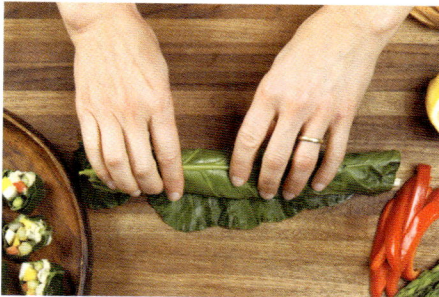

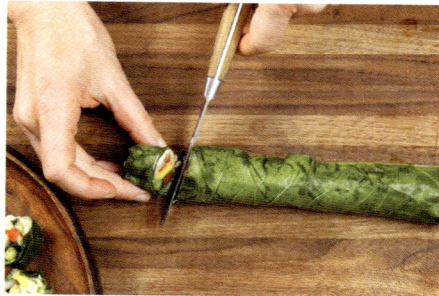

BROWN RICE WRAPS WITH BABY SPINACH AND MUSHROOMS

I've never liked bready wraps. Engine 2 Brown Rice Tortillas, however, make the best, crispy, delicious wraps. But you have to warm the wraps before working with them or they will crumble. If Engine 2 brand wraps are not available to you, any wrap made without oil will work. You can fill your favorite wraps with anything: chopped tomatoes, frozen corn, grilled zucchini and onions, leftover rice and beans, mango, cooked greens, etc.

INGREDIENTS:

8 to 10 ounces mushrooms, sliced, or 1 large portobello mushroom, sliced

2 tablespoons balsamic vinegar

2 brown-rice wraps

4 tablespoons (or more) hummus prepared without oil or tahini

2 green onions, chopped

½ cup fresh cilantro, parsley, basil, or mint, chopped

2 large handfuls of baby spinach or other greens (kale, Swiss chard, etc.), cooked and well drained (see page 23)

INSTRUCTIONS:

Preheat the oven to 450°F. Line a baking sheet with parchment paper.

Heat a large frying pan over medium heat. Place the mushrooms perfectly flat on the surface of the pan and cook without turning for 5 minutes. Sprinkle the mushrooms with about 1 tablespoon of the balsamic vinegar. Flip them and continue cooking briefly, until they are brown and the liquid has mostly evaporated.

In a small frying pan, warm each brown rice wrap, one at a time, over medium heat for about 30 seconds per side. (This step is key if you are using brown rice wraps, as this makes them flexible enough to roll.) Spread the hummus onto one side of the warmed wrap, then top with green onions, cilantro, and mushrooms. Stack a handful or two of spinach on top of the mushrooms. Finally, sprinkle the filling with about ½ tablespoon of the balsamic vinegar.

Carefully fold the wraps into sausagelike shapes. Use both hands as you roll the wrap and keep stuffing all the ingredients inside as you roll.

With a very sharp knife, cut the wraps in half on an angle. Gently place the wraps on the parchment-lined baking sheet. Bake for 10 minutes, until brown and crispy.

Serve immediately. These are messy but good eating!

WRAPS!

My mom used to take anything (anything!) we had for dinner at night and throw it inside a whole wheat pita for my dad's lunch the next day. Without a syllable of complaint he would head off to the clinic in the morning with a football-size pita for lunch. Sometimes the pita was stuffed with veggie lasagna and green beans, or spaghetti and salad, or beans and rice with salsa, or mashed potatoes with gravy and asparagus. Some days it might have just been broccoli florets and hummus. Anything could have been stuffed into those pitas. That is the inspiration behind our wraps—anything can get rolled into a wrap. We have a few ideas here for you, but please do not feel limited to these ideas.

THE BASIC IDEA IS:

1. Lay out a wrap.

2. Layer on the goodness.

3. Roll it up.

4. Eat it up or . . .

5. Heat it up! Toast the filled wrap in the oven at 450°F for 8 to 10 minutes, or until the outside gets crispy or browned to your liking. *Then* eat it up!

SOME FILLING SUGGESTIONS:

1. **Veggie and Cheeze Wrap**—spread a layer of Lemony Cheezy Sauce (page 112) on a wrap; top with sliced lettuce, tomatoes, strips of kale, and sprouts; and roll it up.

2. **The Berlin**—spread a layer of hummus on a wrap; top with a layer of kale pieces (no stems), a layer of sauerkraut, and a squirt of mustard; and roll it up. We recommend heating up this one.

3. **The Matthew**—start with a layer of brown rice, then a layer of Matt's Sofrito Black Beans (page 209), then a layer of fresh spinach, and roll it up. We recommend serving this with salsa of your choice. We love it with Down Under Cranberry Salsa (page 121) or Mango-Lime Salsa (page 120).

4. **Hot Stuff**—lay down a layer of Chile Rellenos (page 218) covered with a sprinkling of hot sauce; then roll it up, toast it, and serve with more hot sauce and Pico de Gallo (page 119) or Mango-Lime Salsa (page 120).

5. **Plain Jane Wrap**—spread a layer of hummus first, top with raw or cooked vegetables, then roll it up.

6. **Luscious Caramelized Onion Wrap**—start with a layer of Caramelized Onion Hummus (page 104), then Roasted Red Peppers (page 24), then butter lettuce and tomato slices, and roll it up. Yummy, yummy.

7. **Dal Wrap**—start with a layer of Singapore Dal (page 215), then a layer of chopped bok choy, greens, or lettuce, and finally chopped green onions, and roll it up.

8. **Emergency Wrap**—spread a layer of mustard on a wrap; then top with lettuce and raw or cooked cucumbers, tomatoes, green onions, celery, and/or beets (or any vegetables you like!), and roll it up!

9. **Rainbow Wrap**—spread a layer of hummus on a wrap, top with a mixture of cubes of cooked beets, cooked cauliflower, cooked broccoli, carrots, red bell peppers, and blueberries (yes!), and roll it up.

10. **Parallel Universe Wrap**—spread a layer of hummus on a wrap; then add a layer of steamed greens. Repeat that layering pattern three times, then roll it up, heat it up, or eat it up. Up to you.

11. **Italian Wrap**—fill a wrap with last night's lasagna, spaghetti, or penne pasta with Besto Pesto (page 126), add a little spinach, then roll it up and there's your lunch. Warm or cold, your choice.

12. **Tex-Mex Wrap**—spread a layer of vegetarian, no-oil refried beans on a wrap, top with cooked brown rice and black beans mixed together, then add red bell peppers, corn, and green onions. Roll it up and heat it up before you serve it with Mango-Lime Salsa (page 120), Pico de Gallo (page 119), or Pomegranate Salsa (page 124).

13. **Asian Wrap**—lay Pacific Rim Soba Noodles (page 190) on the wrap horizontally, add a layer of Light Asian Slaw (page 163), then roll it up.

14. **BBQ Wrap**—spread a layer Caramelized Onion Hummus (page 104) on a wrap, add a layer of cooked brown rice, Sautéed Mushrooms cooked with barbecue sauce (see Variation 2, page 28), and steamed kale, then roll it up. Wow. Yum.

ROCKIN' SPRING ROLLS

MAKES 6 TO 10 SPRING ROLLS
(DEPENDING ON HOW MUCH STUFFING YOU ADD!)

We love the fresh spring rolls in Thai restaurants. To our delight, we find spring rolls are also surprisingly easy and fun to make. Fill them with whatever you have or buy things you think might be good. Just cut everything into thin strips. These rolls are delicious dipped in a light plum sauce or low-sodium tamari. My dad even puts hummus on his, to everyone's horror. We buy the brown rice paper wrappers online, but look in the Asian section of the grocery store. The wrappers tear easily but are also tougher than you might think.

INGREDIENTS:

12 fresh mint leaves

12 fresh basil leaves

Brown rice noodles (we use Annie Chun's Thin Maifun Rice Noodles), prepared as directed on the package

½ cucumber, peeled (if desired), seeded, and cut lengthwise into thin strips

½ red bell pepper, seeded and cut lengthwise into thin strips

1 to 2 carrots, cut lengthwise into thin strips

2 green onions, cut lengthwise into thin strips

2 stalks bok choy, cut lengthwise into thin strips

1 small mango, pitted, peeled, and cut lengthwise into thin strips

2 cups fresh spinach leaves

Brown rice spring roll wrappers (we use Happy Pho brand)

Light plum sauce, low-sodium tamari, or sauce of your choice

INSTRUCTIONS:

Fill a flat dish with ½ inch or so of water. Have two more plates nearby: one for constructing the spring rolls and one for holding your beautiful spring roll creations. Then, set up the prepared filling items in your preferred order near the water-filled plate. Our preferred order is: mint and basil leaves, cooked noodles, cucumbers, bell peppers, carrots, green onions, bok choy, mango, and spinach leaves.

Remove one rice paper wrapper and submerge it in the water until it becomes flexible enough to wrap, about a minute—if you leave it too long in the water, it gets too soggy and it will tear; if you don't leave it in long enough it will be too dry and snap. You will soon find the

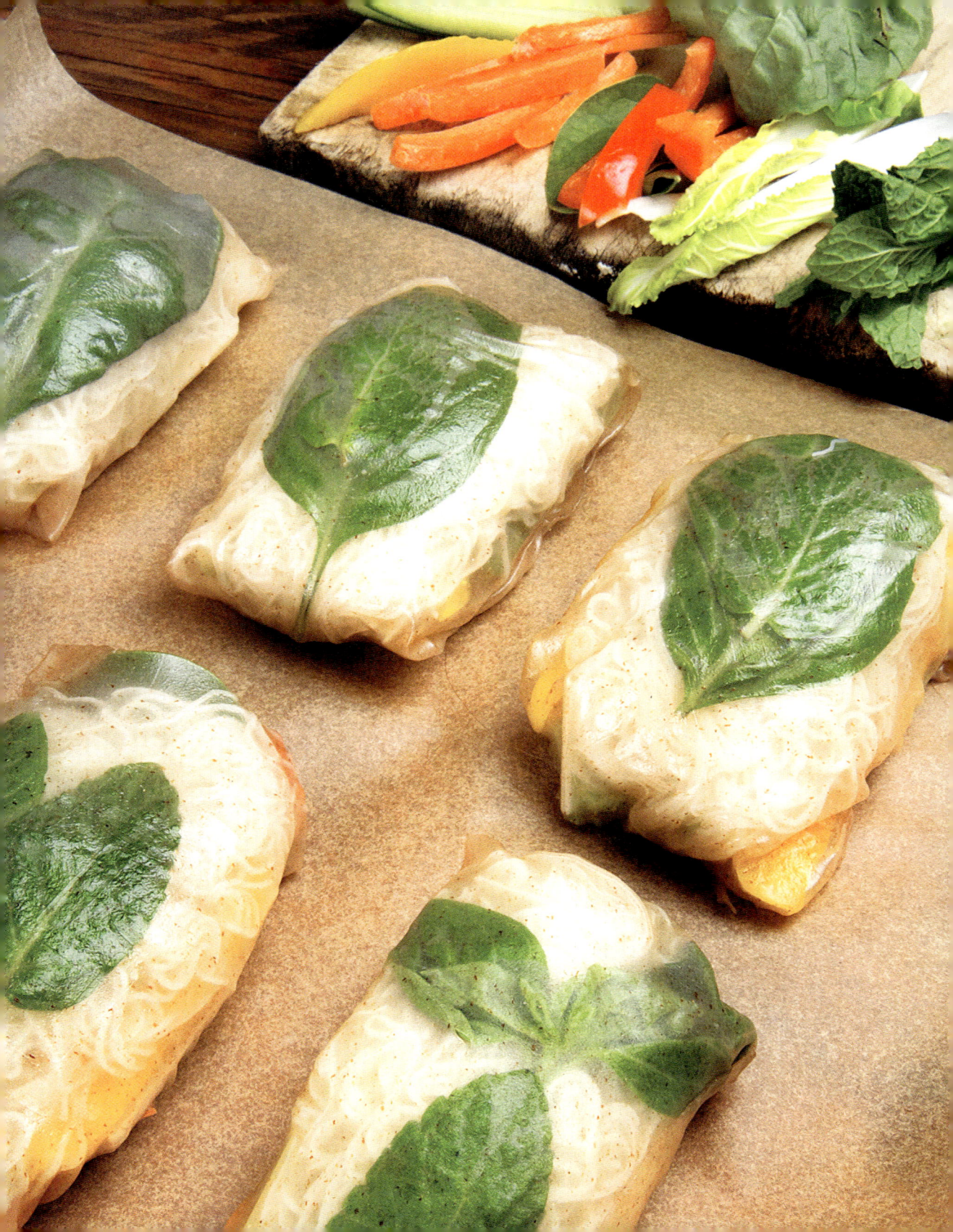

perfect amount of time needed for soaking. Gently remove the wrapper with both hands and place it on the constructing plate. It is okay if this plate gets a bit wet—it actually keeps the wrapper from sticking as you construct the spring rolls.

Now that it is time to construct the spring rolls, treat the wrapper like a face. In the center line of the nose, place a fresh mint leaf and a basil leaf, then in the same vertical space of the nose add a small clump of noodles, a line of cucumber, bell pepper, carrots, green onion, bok choy, and mango, and top with some fresh spinach leaves. All should be in the center of the face like a large nose.

Carefully fold one side (one cheek of the face) over the top of the vegetables as far as it will go. Then fold up the bottom (the chin of the face) over the side you just folded. Fold the top (forehead of the face) over the rolled side; then roll the last side (the last cheek of the face) over the vegetables as far as possible and form into a tight sausage shape. Place the formed spring roll on the third (empty) plate, and repeat with the remaining wrappers and filling.

Serve immediately, with whatever sauce you wish alongside for dipping.

LUNCH ON THE ROAD

You can make this on the road or any bagel shop can whip it up for you.

INGREDIENTS:

- 1 whole wheat bagel
- 2 tablespoons mustard, your favorite
- 1 tomato, sliced
- 4 lettuce leaves

INSTRUCTIONS:

Slice the bagel in half, spread mustard on both sides, and add generous amounts of tomato and lettuce. Eat as an open-faced or closed sandwich. It's a winner as a quick bite on the road.

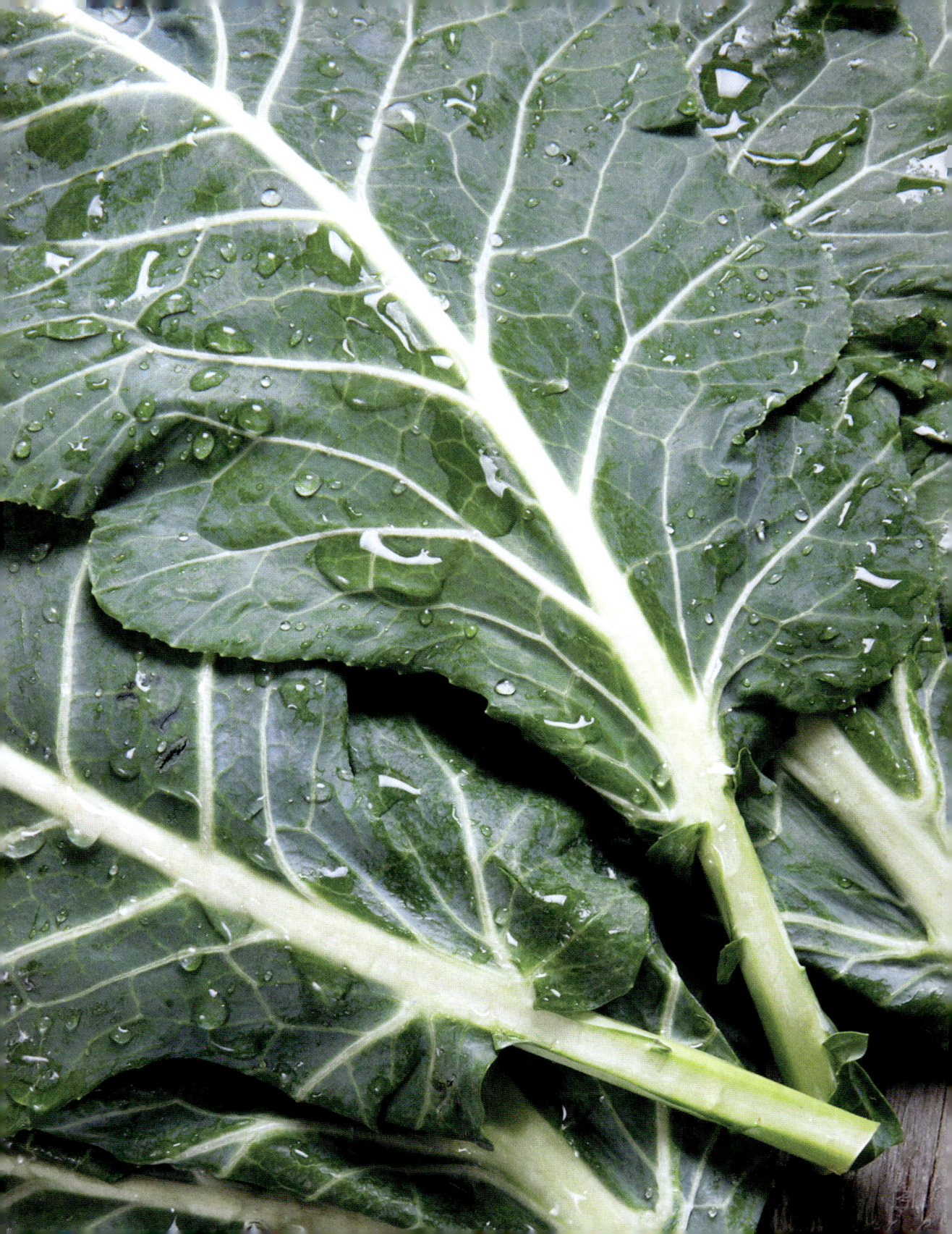

SOUPS

We absolutely *love* soup—especially thick soups! As my husband says, "Soup is best when it is thick enough to walk on." (But if you don't share our preference and find any of these soups too thick, you can always thin them with vegetable broth or water.)

A bowl of soup, full of greens, is part of almost every lunch for us. And when served with a big salad and bread, soup also makes a wonderful dinner. If you make a big batch of soup, every time you reheat it, *add more greens*. They tend to disappear. You can easily add greens to a hot soup by putting some spinach in your bowl first before adding your soup. The spinach will wilt from just the heat of the soup. Or add chopped Swiss chard or bok choy to a simmering pot of soup and allow it to cook a few minutes before serving. If you want to use kale and collards, they'll need to cook at least 5 to 10 minutes in a soup before they are ready. Depending on the final soup color, use the darker Kitchen Basics unsalted vegetable stock or the lighter Pacific low-sodium vegetable broth or even water. When not using salt, vegetable broth helps add flavor.

Luxuriate in the variety of soups in this section and be sure you fill whatever soup you make with greens.

RED LENTIL AND DILL SOUP WITH MINT

This soup is adapted from a recipe of Kate Sherwood's in the Nutrition Action *newsletter. The red lentils, bits of tomato, and all the greens combine with the mint and dill to give the soup a well-rounded flavor. Nothing beats using fresh mint if you can find it. The twelve ounces of spinach seems like a lot, but it vanishes so quickly. Be bold!*

INGREDIENTS:

12 cloves garlic, minced

8 green onions, chopped (about 1 cup)

1 (15-ounce) can no-salt-added diced tomatoes

¼ cup fresh mint, chopped, or 1 teaspoon dried

1 teaspoon dried oregano

8 cups vegetable broth

2 cups red lentils

1 large yam, preferably a garnet yam, peeled, if desired, and cubed

1 cup orange juice

8 sprigs fresh dill, chopped (about ¼ cup)

12 ounces fresh spinach or other greens

Zest of 1 lemon

3 tablespoons lemon juice

1 teaspoon freshly ground black pepper

2 tablespoons balsamic vinegar

INSTRUCTIONS:

In a soup pot, stir-fry the garlic and green onions in water, wine, or vegetable broth, for about 2 minutes, until they begin to wilt.

Add the diced tomatoes, mint, and oregano, and cook, stirring often, for 2 minutes more.

Add the broth, lentils, yam, and orange juice, and bring to a boil. Cover, reduce the heat to low, and simmer until the yams are tender and the lentils soft but not mushy, about 15 minutes

With an immersion blender, blend the soup to the consistency you like, right in the pot. Alternatively, carefully transfer half of the soup to a food processor and process it until you have the texture you desire. Try to leave some whole bits of tomato and sweet potato. This soup is nice if it's a little chunky.

Stir in the dill, spinach, lemon zest, lemon juice, pepper, and vinegar, and cook for a few minutes more. Serve hot.

TIP:

If you want to use greens other than spinach, cook them first or add them to the soup earlier as it cooks, so they have time to soften.

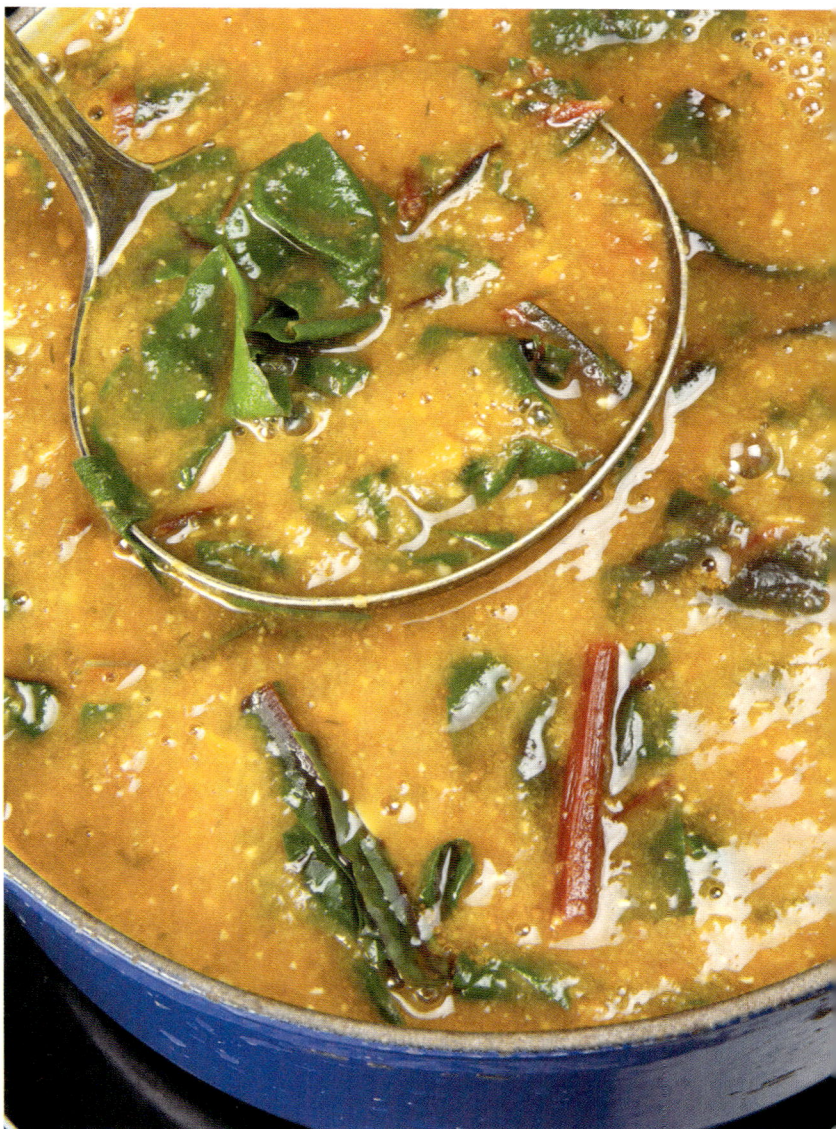

TARRAZAN SOUP

This soup is king of the plant-strong jungle. It has a subtle tarragon taste, which is balanced nicely by the slightly sweet yams. It cooks in two stages so that the peas become creamy while the yams and onions keep some of their texture. Fresh tarragon makes all *the difference. This soup is perfect for a great lunch or a delicious dinner with bread and a great big green salad. After eating this soup, you will want to swing from limb to limb, just like Tarzan!*

INGREDIENTS:

8 cups vegetable broth or water

2 cups green split peas or yellow split peas

1 bay leaf

½ teaspoon dry mustard

1 large red onion, chopped (2 to 2½ cups)

1 large or 2 medium yams, peeled, if desired, and diced (6 to 7 cups)

½ cup fresh tarragon (about ¾ ounce plastic container), or 2 teaspoons dried

½ to 1 teaspoon freshly ground black pepper

1 to 2 tablespoons balsamic vinegar, to taste

2 baby bok choy, diced (2 cups)

1 cup fresh cilantro or parsley, chopped

INSTRUCTIONS:

Put the broth, split peas, bay leaf, and mustard in a soup pot. Bring to a boil, cover, and reduce the heat to maintain a simmer. Simmer for 40 minutes, until the peas begin to break down.

Add the onion, yams, and tarragon, stir, bring back to a boil, then cover and simmer for 20 to 30 minutes more, or until the yams are tender and the peas are creamy.

Add the pepper, vinegar, bok choy, and cilantro. Stir and simmer for about 3 minutes so the bok choy has time to soften.

Mash some of the yams against the side of the pot with a wooden spoon for a smoother soup. We like it best when about half the yams have been mashed.

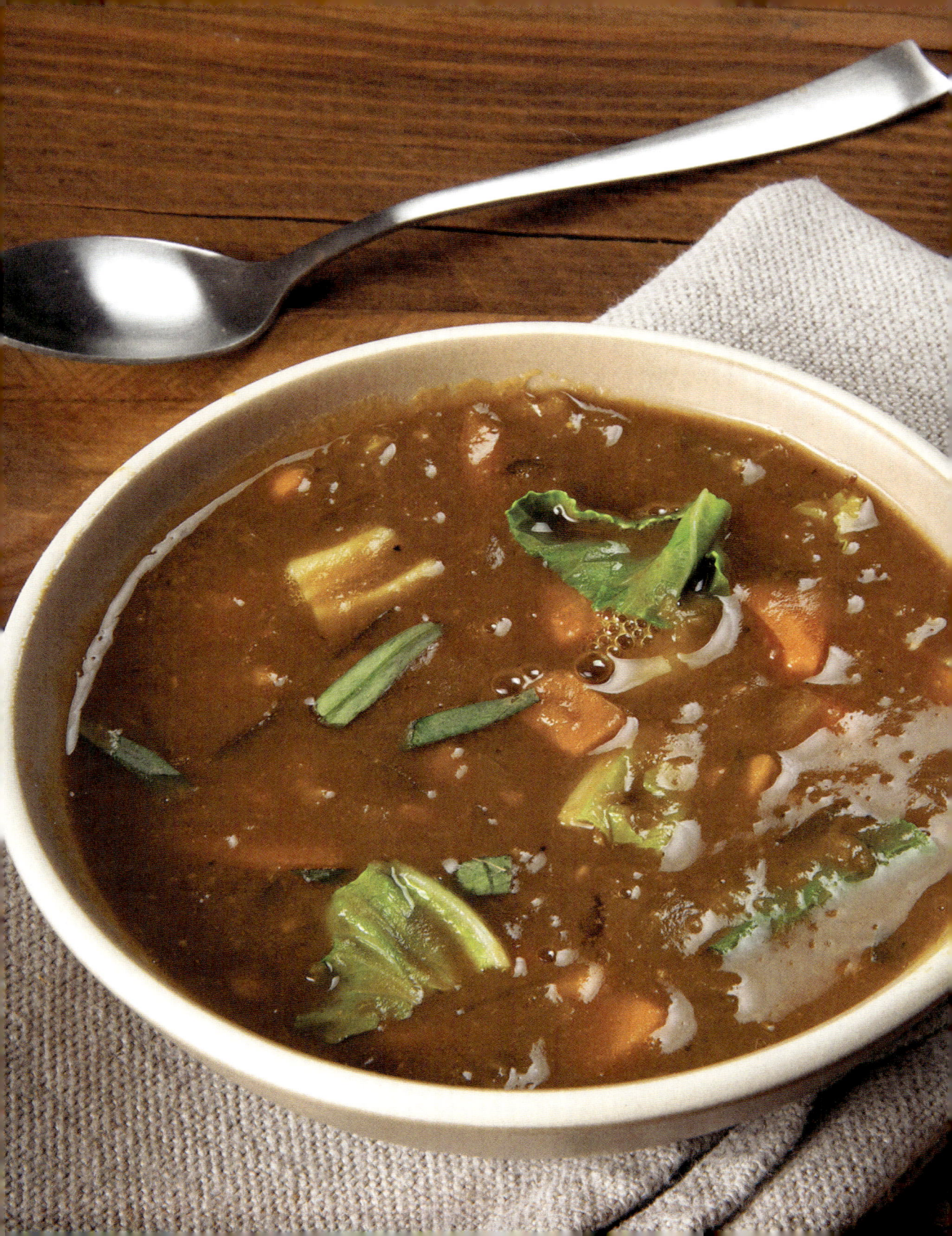

ENDOTHELIUM-ENHANCING BEET SOUP

SERVES 4

This is a favorite cold summer soup for us. And also an endothelium enhancer! Yes, beets help endothelial cells dance! This is a gorgeous deep red color made with red beets, but if you use Chioggia beets, it is a lovely pale pink. The beets can be boiled, baked, or steamed until tender for this soup.

INGREDIENTS:

1 bunch beets (about 3 medium), trimmed, cooked, and peeled

1 orange, peeled and sectioned

2 tablespoons grated lemon zest

2 tablespoons lemon juice

2 tablespoons mint, or to taste, plus 4 mint leaves, for serving

Freshly ground black pepper

INSTRUCTIONS:

Put the beets in a blender and blend until smooth. Add the orange sections, lemon zest, and lemon juice, and blend some more. Be sure to scrape down the sides of the blender.

Add the mint and pepper, and blend well again. Serve with a mint leaf on top of each serving.

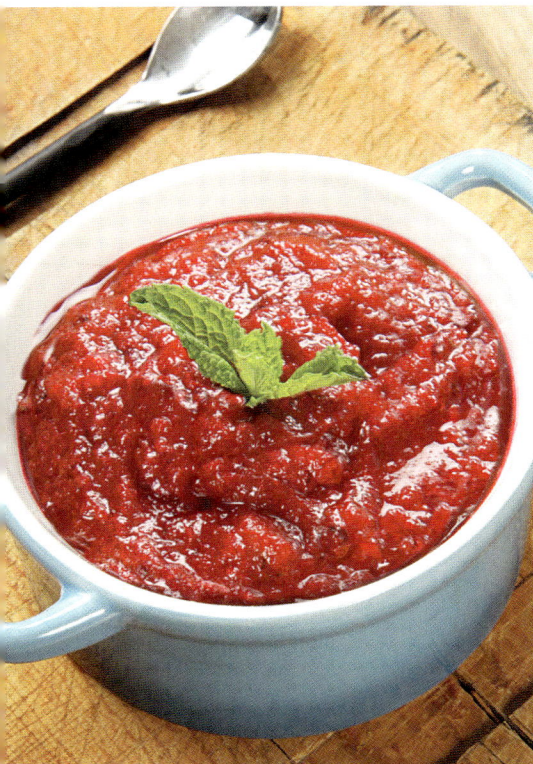

GEORGIE'S SOUP

We have a special feeling about this soup because while I was making it, we heard the exciting news that our son Zeb's wife, Polly, was pregnant. Our ninth grandchild on the way! (They named her Georgie.) So this is a special soup. And oh my, it is good! Use less liquid and it could be a topping for rice or potatoes. You might want to consider making it the day before you want to serve it, since it just gets better the longer it sits.

INGREDIENTS:

- 1 large sweet onion, chopped
- 1 large leek, white and as much of the green as possible, chopped
- 1 large fennel bulb, trimmed and chopped
- 16 ounces mushrooms, sliced
- 2 teaspoons dried thyme, or 2 tablespoons fresh thyme leaves
- 1 cup red lentils
- 6 cups vegetable broth
- 2 medium white or sweet potatoes, cubed
- 1 cup shredded carrots
- ½ teaspoon freshly ground black pepper
- ⅛ teaspoon cayenne pepper
- 1 tablespoon balsamic vinegar
- 1 cup fresh cilantro, chopped, or 1 bunch Swiss chard or spinach, chopped

INSTRUCTIONS:

In a soup pot, combine the onion, leek, and fennel, and stir-fry over medium heat in a bit of water or broth until limp and beginning to brown. Add a little more liquid as necessary to prevent burning. This may take 10 minutes. Keep stirring.

Add the mushrooms and thyme, and continue to cook, stirring, for 5 minutes, until the mushrooms begin to soften.

Add the lentils, vegetable broth, and potatoes. Cover, reduce the heat to low, and simmer for 20 minutes, or until the lentils have begun to dissolve and the potatoes are tender.

Add the carrots, black pepper, cayenne, vinegar, and cilantro, and cook for a few minutes more. Serve immediately, or refrigerate in an airtight container until ready to serve—the flavors will continue to develop. Reheat before serving.

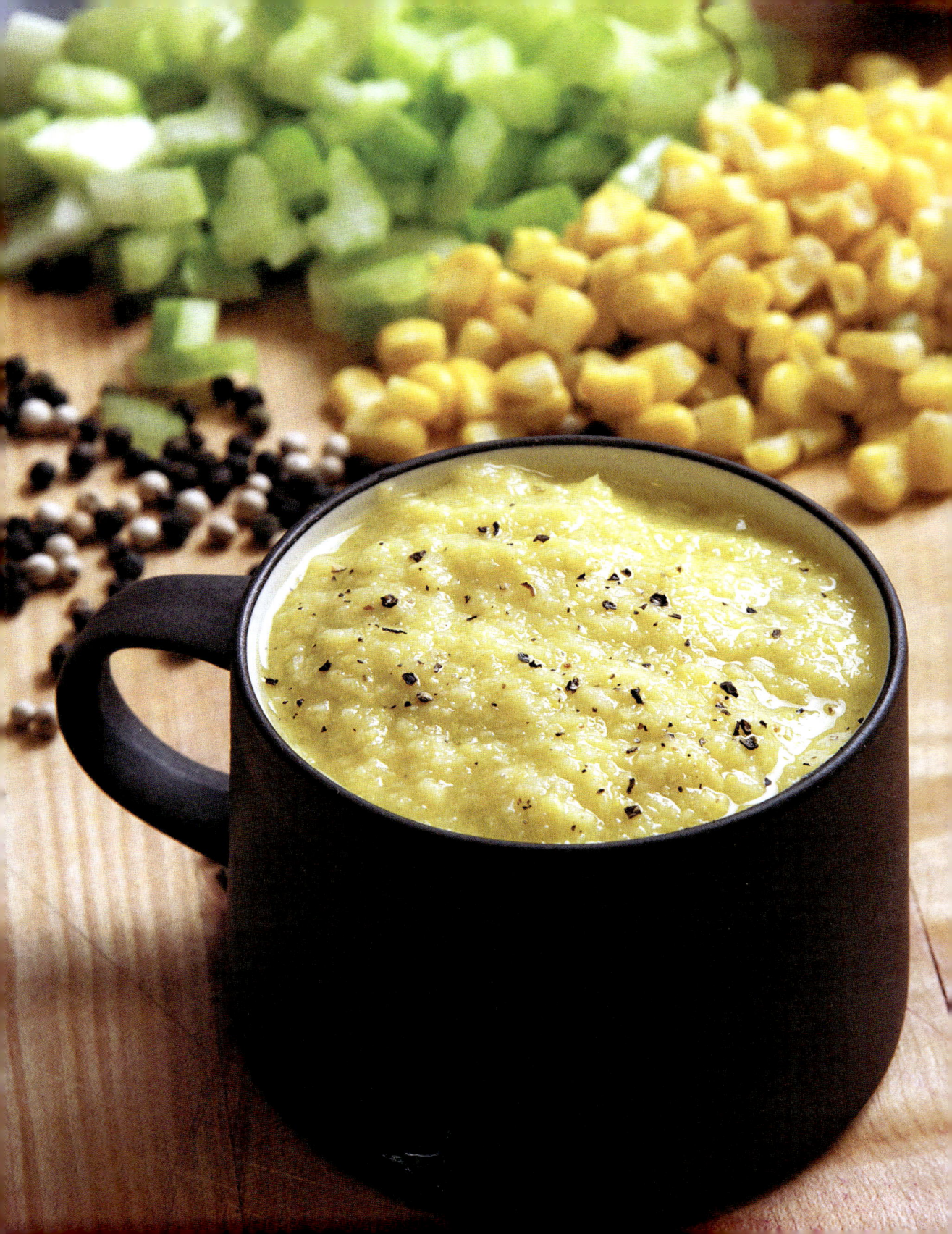

OBERLIN CORN AND SHALLOT CHOWDER

This creamy, thick corn chowder was served to us by the talented Chef Wayne Jacob at Kendal at Oberlin. We had a 4:30 dinner before our talk at 6:00, and what a feast it was—beginning with this delicious chowder, which arrived in little black cups. Everyone raved! The color of this soup is so vibrant. Chef Wayne noted that this is because the corn is not cooked to death, just heated briefly so the corn really shines. Pacific's low-sodium vegetable broth is light enough in color to keep the soup a bright yellow. We actually prefer using vegetable broth over wine when we make this soup.

INGREDIENTS:

- 1 shallot, chopped (½ cup)
- 1 large stalk celery, chopped (½ cup)
- 2 cups vegetable broth (we recommend Pacific brand low-sodium)
- 1 (16-ounce) bag frozen sweet corn, thawed, or kernels from 5 to 6 ears fresh corn (sweet corn makes all the difference here)
- 1 tablespoon white balsamic vinegar (optional)
- ½ teaspoon freshly ground black pepper

INSTRUCTIONS:

Put shallot, celery, and broth in a medium saucepan, bring to a boil, then reduce the heat to maintain a simmer and cook until the vegetables are soft, about 10 minutes.

Transfer the shallot mixture to a food processor, add the corn, and process until smooth.

Add the balsamic vinegar, return the soup to the pan, and heat until just simmering. Watch closely—do not overcook the soup or it will lose its vibrant color. Remove from the heat, add the pepper, and serve.

POLLY'S LENTIL SOUP

This is a thick and delicious soup that just seems to get better each day. Our daughter-in-law Polly first gave us the idea. We have used a version of it at the monthly Cleveland Clinic Wellness Institute seminars, and here we have added our special touches. Add kale as indicated in the recipe or 10 minutes before the soup is ready so that it stays green, or cook it separately and put some in the bottom of each soup bowl as you serve it, as we do at the Wellness Institute. We usually double the amount of kale.

INGREDIENTS:

2 cups (1 pound) French lentils (small, green)

1 large onion (2 to 3 cups), chopped

1 large leek (2 to 3 cups), chopped

6 cloves garlic, chopped

1½ teaspoons black pepper

1½ teaspoons dried thyme or 1 tablespoon fresh thyme

1 teaspoon cumin

3 cups carrots (about 6), chopped

3 cups celery (about 6 stalks), chopped

10 cups vegetable broth or water

8 ounces mushrooms, sliced

2 to 3 medium red potatoes, diced ½ inch thick (2 cups)

6 ounces tomato paste

1 bunch (6 to 8 cups) kale, stripped and chopped (including stems)

4 tablespoons balsamic vinegar to taste

Hot sauce, to taste (Cholulu recommended)

INSTRUCTIONS:

Place lentils in a large soup pot, cover with 2 cups of boiling water, and let sit for 15 minutes. Drain, return to the soup pot, and set aside.

In a large frying pan over medium-high heat, cook the onions, leeks, and garlic a few minutes until they begin to soften.

Reduce the heat to medium-low and add the pepper, thyme, and cumin. Stir and cook for about 15 minutes, or until the onions are translucent. Add liquid or vegetable broth as needed.

Add the carrots and celery and cook about 10 minutes, or until beginning to soften.

Transfer vegetables to the large soup pot with lentils.

Add the vegetable broth, mushrooms, potatoes, tomato paste, and kale, and bring to a boil.

Reduce heat to simmer and cook, covered, 25 minutes or until the lentils are tender. Stir occasionally.

Add balsamic vinegar, stir, and serve with whole-grain bread and a big salad, and you have the perfect lunch or dinner.

We love this soup's thickness, but if it's too thick for you, add vegetable broth or water. Don't forget that sprinkle of Cholulu hot sauce, which is especially good with this soup.

CITRUS GAZPACHO

We have always loved gazpacho! In Prevent and Reverse Heart Disease *and* My Beef with Meat, *my mom and I included our favorite gazpacho recipes. But here she adds a new twist—Citrus Gazpacho.*

Nothing is as refreshing on a hot summer day as this soup. The oranges add a delicious new taste to a traditional gazpacho. Find a tomato juice low in sodium. R.W. Knudsen Very Veggie is good (35 mg sodium per 8 ounces), as is Kagome Sweet Summer Tomato Juice (100 mg sodium per 8 ounces).

INGREDIENTS:

2 to 3 oranges

2 tomatoes, cored and chopped

1 small cucumber, peeled (optional), seeded, and chopped

½ green bell pepper, seeded and finely chopped

1 small shallot, finely chopped

1 to 2 cloves garlic, minced

1 tablespoon chopped fresh basil, plus more for serving, or 1 teaspoon dried basil

8 ounces low-sodium tomato juice

1 to 2 tablespoons red wine vinegar or balsamic vinegar

Pinch of cayenne pepper

⅛ teaspoon freshly ground black pepper

Chopped green onions, for serving (optional)

INSTRUCTIONS:

Peel the oranges with a knife, removing the skin and white pith. Working over a large bowl, remove the orange sections from between the membrane, letting them fall into the bowl; then squeeze all juice out of what remains into the bowl. With scissors or a knife, cut each section into 2 or 3 bite-size pieces.

Add the tomatoes, cucumber, bell pepper, shallot, garlic, basil, tomato juice, vinegar, cayenne, and black pepper to the bowl. Stir well, cover, and chill for at least 2 hours or overnight, if possible.

To serve, garnish with additional basil, chopped green onions, or mint.

LIGHT SPRING PEA SOUP

This is really quick to make and so springlike and good. If you love mushrooms, add more. Or feel free to skip them entirely.

INGREDIENTS:

1 large onion, chopped

16 ounces frozen peas

4 cups vegetable stock (we recommend Pacific brand low-sodium)

⅔ cup fresh mint, chopped

8 ounces mushrooms, chopped

1 tablespoon balsamic vinegar

½ teaspoon freshly ground black pepper

3 to 4 green onions, chopped (about ½ cup)

INSTRUCTIONS:

In a soup pot, cook the onions over medium heat until they are limp and just beginning to brown. Add a few drops of liquid as necessary if the pan gets dry.

Add the peas, stock, and mint. Bring to a boil, cover, reduce heat to maintain a simmer, and cook for 3 to 4 minutes.

In a frying pan or wok, spread out the mushrooms and cook over medium heat, without turning, for 4 to 5 minutes. Sprinkle the mushrooms with the balsamic vinegar, stir, and continue cooking for a few minutes more, until browned.

Blend the peas with an immersion blender right in the pot. Alternatively, working in batches, transfer the pea mixture to a food processor and process until as smooth as desired.

Add the mushrooms and pepper to the soup, stir, sprinkle with the green onions, and enjoy!

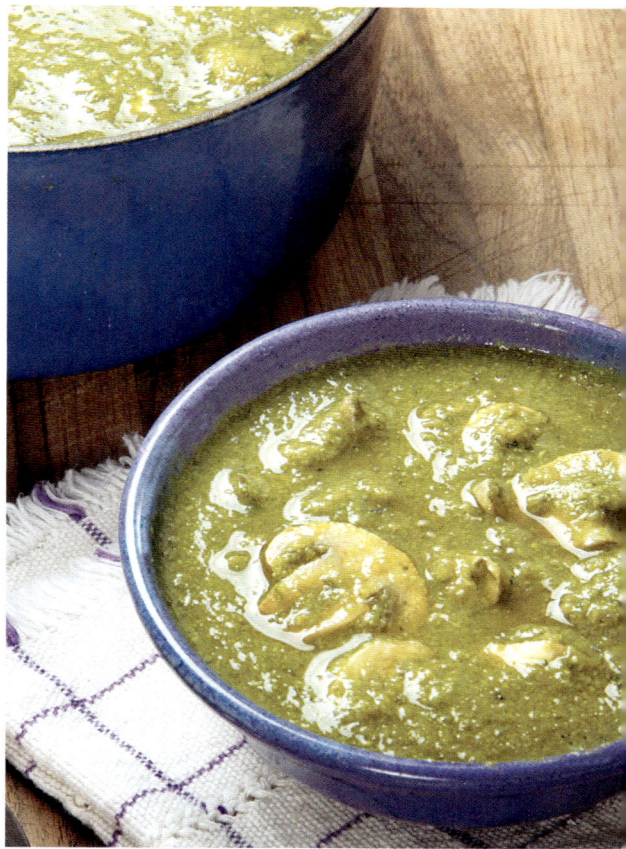

MIDDLE EASTERN CHICKPEA STEW

Chef Martin Oswald, owner of the Pyramid Bistro in Aspen, Colorado, is the rock star of vegan cooking. We were fortunate to have experienced two of his meals in a row. Every bite was perfection. His chickpea soup was amazing, and he generously shared the recipe. Normally when I use anyone's recipe I have to adapt it, but this is not *true of anything Chef Oswald makes. He says you can substitute the veggies below with any bean, lentil, greens, or other vegetable.*

INGREDIENTS:

1 medium onion, diced

2 tablespoons peeled, minced fresh ginger

2 cloves garlic, chopped

1 tablespoon curry powder

½ teaspoon ground turmeric

1 teaspoon ground coriander

½ teaspoon ground cardamom

1 teaspoon ground cinnamon

½ teaspoon ground cloves

½ cup fresh orange juice

6 cups vegetable stock

1 (15-ounce) can chickpeas, drained and rinsed

1 cup green lentils

1 (14.5-ounce) can crushed Cento San Marzano tomatoes

1 large sweet potato, diced (peeling optional)

2 tablespoons red wine vinegar

2 cups Swiss chard

Pinch of cayenne pepper

1 cup fresh cilantro, chopped

Brown rice or quinoa, for serving (optional)

INSTRUCTIONS:

In a large stockpot, combine the onions, ginger, and garlic, and cook over medium-high heat until tender, about 5 minutes.

Add the curry powder, turmeric, coriander, cardamom, cinnamon, and cloves, and stir for about 15 seconds. The spices will stick, so add the orange juice and stir. This will deglaze the pan and coat everything with the flavors of the spices.

Add the stock, chickpeas, lentils, tomatoes, and sweet potato, and bring to a boil. Reduce heat to maintain a gentle simmer, cover, and cook, stirring occasionally, until the lentils and sweet potatoes are tender, about 25 minutes.

Add the vinegar, Swiss chard, and cayenne, and simmer for 2 minutes more, until the Swiss chard has softened.

Sprinkle the cilantro on top and serve alone or over brown rice or quinoa.

SEMINAR SOUP

This is a delicious way to get lots of colors in one bowl. Also, we serve this at the monthly Prevent and Reverse Heart Disease seminars at the Cleveland Clinic Wellness Institute because it is awesomely delicious. At the seminars instead of using spinach as a green of choice, we place a little nest of cooked kale in the bottom of each soup bowl. Any greens will work. Just be sure to include them!

INGREDIENTS:

1 large sweet onion, chopped

7 cloves garlic, chopped

4 stalks celery, chopped (about 2 cups)

4 carrots, chopped (about 2 cups)

1 large sweet potato, peeled, if desired, and chopped

6 cups vegetable broth

1 teaspoon Mrs. Dash garlic and herb

½ teaspoon freshly ground black pepper

6 cups frozen sweet corn, divided (sweet corn makes *all* the difference here)

6 cups fresh spinach, or 1 (16-ounce) package frozen whole-leaf spinach (not chopped)

1 bunch cilantro or parsley, chopped (about 1½ cups)

2 tablespoons balsamic vinegar

INSTRUCTIONS:

In a soup pot, cook the onions over high heat for a few minutes, adding broth or water if necessary to prevent sticking. Add the garlic, celery, carrots, sweet potato, and 1 cup of corn, and continue to cook, stirring, until vegetables soften, about 15 minutes.

Add the broth, bring to a boil, then reduce the heat to maintain a simmer and cook until the vegetables are soft, about 15 minutes.

Stir in the Mrs. Dash garlic and herb and pepper.

Blend the soup with an immersion blender until it begins to thicken. Alternatively, transfer the soup, in batches, to a food processor and process to the desired thickness.

Add the remaining corn, spinach, cilantro, and balsamic vinegar and heat until the corn has thawed and warmed through and the spinach has wilted. Serve with a smile!

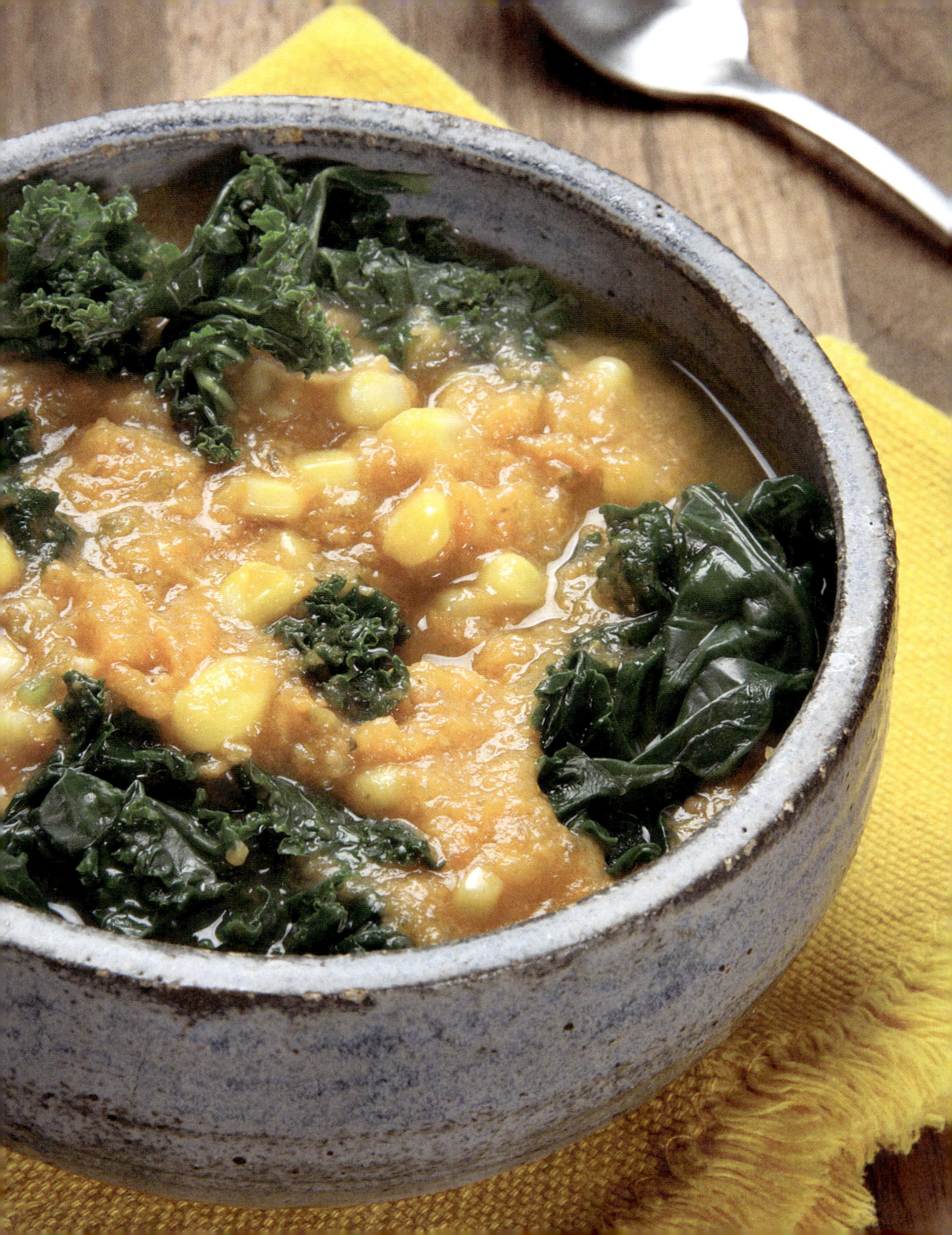

BIG BEAN SOUP

Our daughter-in-law Polly told us about this soup. Since we are lima bean fans, we couldn't resist this interesting combination of big limas and butternut squash! The large limas add a surprise meaty feel and the butternut squash adds a good sweetness. The combination is fabulous! And beautiful. And, oh, those big *beans! Sweet potatoes will work but tend to dominate in taste more than the butternut squash.*

INGREDIENTS:

1 large onion, chopped

1 leek, white and green parts chopped

3 stalks celery, chopped

3 large carrots, cut on an angle into rounds

1 bay leaf

6 cloves garlic, chopped

2 teaspoons dried sage, crumbled

2 teaspoons dried thyme

8 cups vegetable broth

16 ounces dried large lima beans, soaked overnight

1 large butternut squash, or 2 large sweet potatoes

½ teaspoon freshly ground black pepper

½ teaspoon freshly ground white pepper

1 bunch kale, stems removed, leaves torn into bite-size pieces and cooked

1 tablespoon balsamic vinegar, or more to taste

1 cup fresh parsley, chopped

INSTRUCTIONS:

Preheat the oven to 400°F. Line a baking sheet with parchment paper.

In a large soup pot, cook the onions over high heat until they start to wilt and caramelize. Add the leek, celery, carrots, and bay leaf, and continue to cook, stirring, for about 5 minutes, until all the vegetables have softened. Add a little water or broth, if necessary, to keep them from sticking.

Add the garlic, sage, and thyme, and stir for another minute.

Add the broth and lima beans, and bring to a boil. Reduce the heat to low, cover, and simmer for 1 to 1½ hours or until the beans are tender. They should be soft but still have a little crunch in the center. Don't overcook them (but if you do, the soup is still good).

While the soup is cooking, place the butternut squash on the lined baking sheet and poke it a few times with a fork to avoid little explosions. Bake for 1 hour; then remove from the oven, cut in half, remove seeds, and scoop the cooked flesh into a food processor.

Remove about 2 cups of mostly liquid from the pot with the beans and add it to the butternut squash. Process until smooth; then pour the pureed butternut squash into the soup and stir to combine. Add the black and white pepper, and cook until heated through. Remove the bay leaf and add balsamic vinegar and parsley.

To serve, place some cooked kale in each bowl, and fill with the soup. You can also add the kale to the soup, but the kale loses its wonderful color if you don't eat it right away.

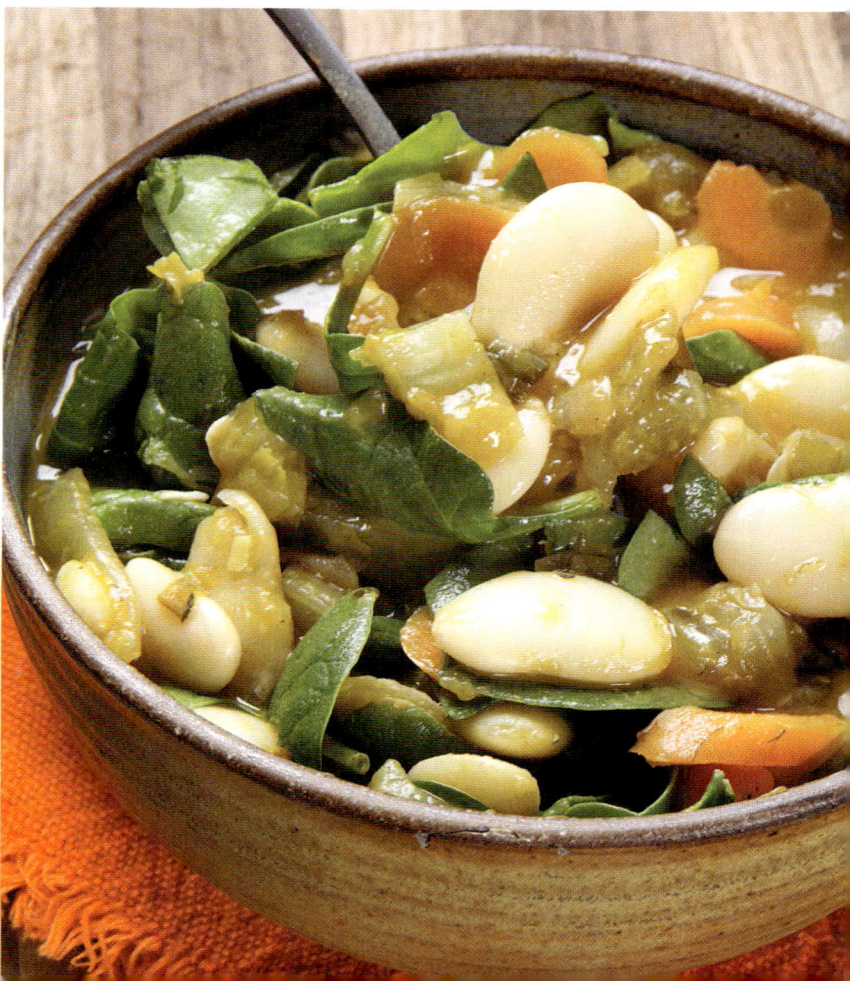

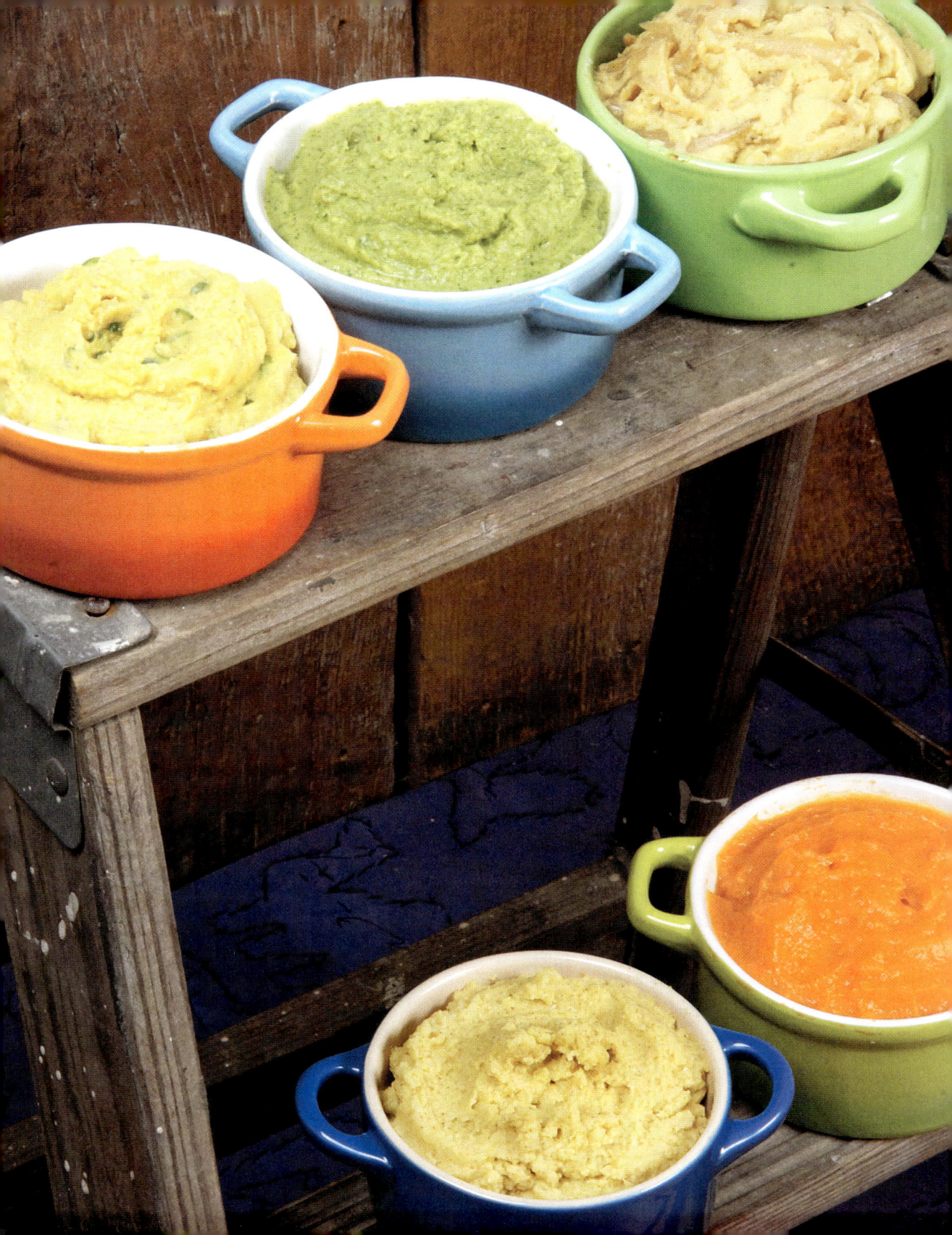

HUMMUS, SAUCES, SPREADS, GRAVY, AND SALSAS

My husband *loves* sauces. There is nothing better than good asparagus or broccoli by itself, but he always goes for a sauce if we have one. And what really makes me frustrated is that he puts on sauce before even trying the dish to see if it needs it!

We have included a few sauces here. They are delicious and add a dose of indulgence to fresh veggie sides, sandwiches, hearty entrées, and more. You don't need nuts to make a luxurious, creamy, plant-based sauce. Our variety here proves it. Wait until you try these!

There is no substitute for cheese, so don't try to find one. All the "vegan" cheeses have oil and casein in them and are simply vegan junk food. Avoid them! But don't worry—you won't miss them for long. Taste is an incredible and malleable sense, and you may well find you enjoy our Lemony Cheezy Sauce even more than dairy cheese, or like me, you may get a taste for some of the magic of nutritional yeast.

When I first tasted nutritional yeast, I didn't like it. Now it is my go-to ingredient when a recipe needs something. Without Jane's cautioning hand, it may have been frighteningly rampant in this book.

OUR HUMMUS

Hummus is your new mayonnaise, your new base for salad dressings, your new spread for sandwiches, your new dip for crackers and veggies, your new best friend. Please note that Our Hummus gets some of its flavor from the mustard and the vinegar in the mustard. If you are not a mustard or vinegar fan, reduce the amount of brown mustard.

INGREDIENTS:

1 (15-ounce) can no-salt-added chickpeas, drained and rinsed

2 large cloves garlic

2 tablespoons fresh lemon juice

1½ tablespoons spicy brown mustard, or to taste

Freshly ground black pepper, to taste

¼ teaspoon salt (optional; we do not use it)

INSTRUCTIONS:

In a food processor, combine the chickpeas, garlic, lemon juice, mustard, pepper to taste, salt (if using), and 2 tablespoons water, and process until uniformly smooth.

Serve immediately or refrigerate until ready to use; refrigerate any leftovers.

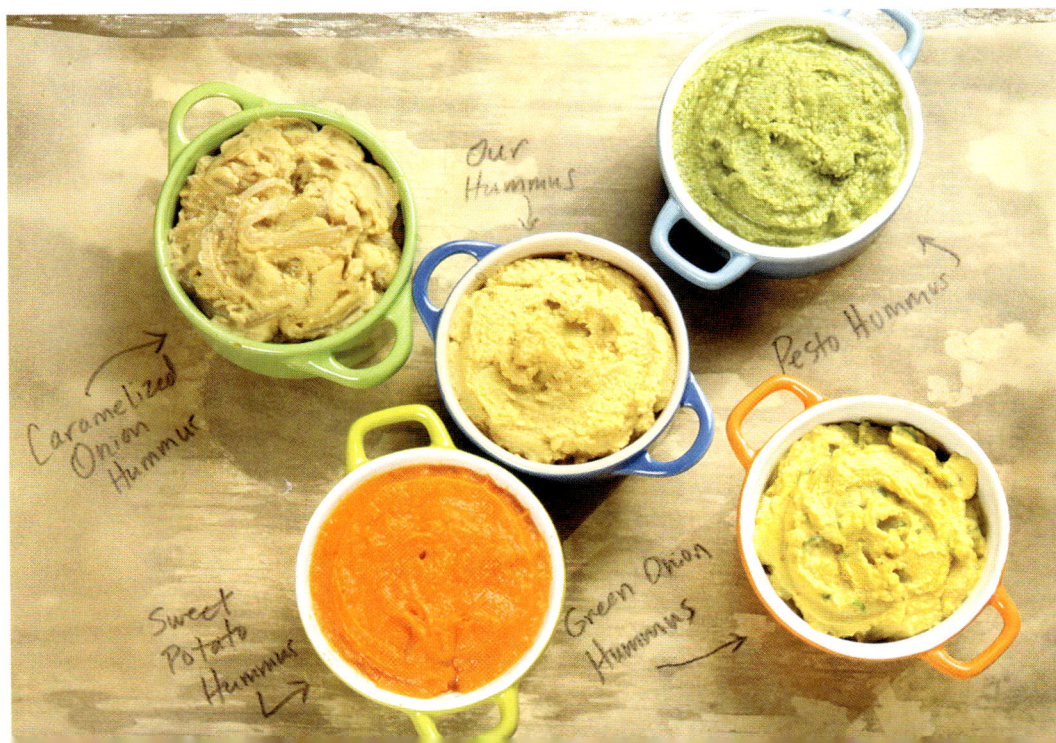

GREEN ONION HUMMUS

This is your new sour cream and chive dip. This spread is delicious on baked potatoes, vegetables, or as a dip or a sandwich spread! And it is the magic inside the Smoky Little Devils (page 132).

INGREDIENTS:

- 1 cup Our Hummus or hummus (page 102) prepared without oil or tahini
- 1 cup chopped green onions (4 to 5)
- 2 teaspoons Dijon mustard, or to taste
- Zest of 1 lemon
- 1½ to 2 tablespoons fresh lemon juice, to taste
- ½ teaspoon ground turmeric

INSTRUCTIONS:

In a small bowl, stir together the hummus, green onions, Dijon mustard, lemon zest, lemon juice, and turmeric. Dollop or spread on immediately or store in an airtight container until ready to use.

VARIATION:

Add fresh dill! Or add vinegar and more lemon juice to make this a salad dressing.

CARAMELIZED ONION HUMMUS

This is just so delicious! We love it on our Tomato Chutney Over Caramelized Onion Hummus Pizza (page 198) and on the Luscious Caramelized Onion Wrap (page 74).

INGREDIENTS:

1 cup Caramelized Onions (page 27)

1 cup Our Hummus (page 102) or hummus prepared without oil or tahini

INSTRUCTIONS:

In a bowl add the onions to the hummus, and stir well. Serve immediately or store in an airtight container until ready to use.

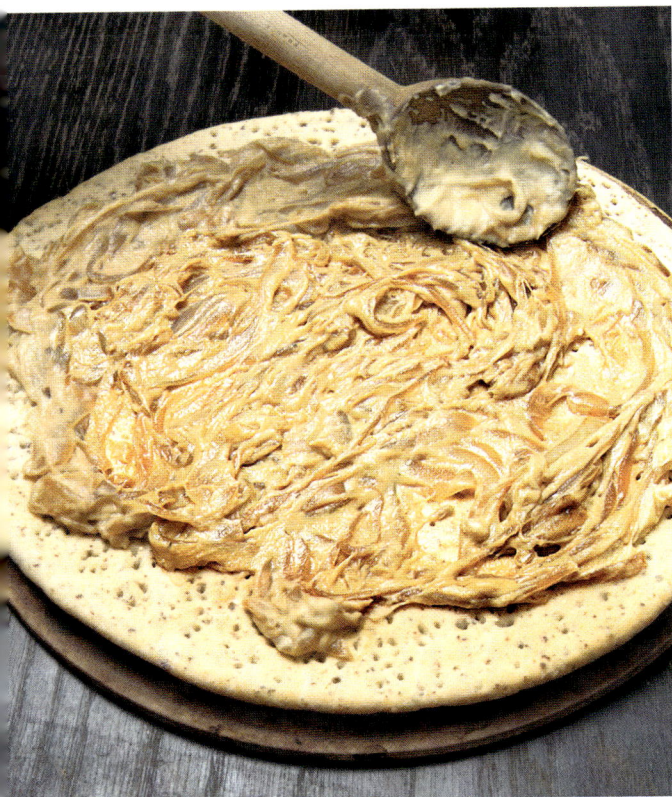

SWEET POTATO HUMMUS

Jim Perko, the creative Cleveland Clinic Wellness Institute chef, created this hummus for the five-hour intensive Prevention and Reversal seminars at the Clinic. It is always a patient favorite when served with crisp, baked pita chips for dipping!

INGREDIENTS:

1 large sweet potato, baked and peeled

1 large red bell pepper, roasted, seeded, and skin removed (page 24), or 1 (4-ounce) jar
    roasted red peppers, drained and blackened skin removed

3 tablespoons fresh lemon juice

1 clove garlic, minced

½ teaspoon ground cumin

Pinch of cayenne pepper

1 tablespoon chopped fresh parsley

INSTRUCTIONS:

In a food processor, combine the sweet potato, roasted peppers, lemon juice, garlic, cumin, and cayenne, and process until smooth. Transfer to a serving bowl, cover, and refrigerate for at least 1 hour.

Sprinkle with the parsley before serving.

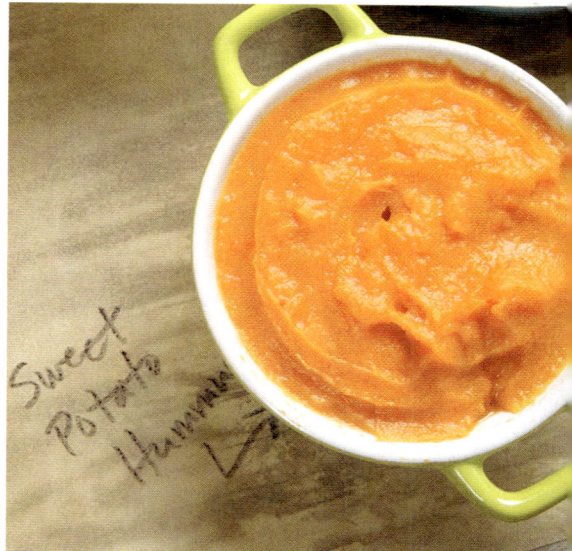

PESTO HUMMUS

This bright green spread is irresistible!

INGREDIENTS:

1 cup Our Hummus (page 102) or hummus prepared without oil or tahini

Zest of 1 lemon

3 tablespoons fresh lemon juice

1 cup packed fresh basil leaves

INSTRUCTIONS:

In a food processor, combine the hummus, lemon zest, lemon juice, and basil, and process until a beautiful, smooth, aromatic pesto hummus appears!

PEAR-APPLE CHUTNEY

Chutney blends ingredients that I would not intuitively put together—yet they are so harmonious and delicious when you do! This is my husband Brian's recipe, which he makes along with a great Indian feast. We love it with Aloo Paratha–Stuffed Indian Tortillas (page 148), Singapore Dal (page 215), and the Dal Wrap (page 74).

INGREDIENTS:

1 pear, unpeeled, chopped

2 apples, unpeeled, chopped

1 teaspoon ground cloves

1 clove garlic, minced

1 teaspoon ground cinnamon

⅓ cup apple cider vinegar

INSTRUCTIONS:

In a saucepan, combine the pear, apples, cloves, garlic, cinnamon, and vinegar. Bring to a boil; then reduce the heat to maintain a simmer and cook for 40 minutes, or until everything is soft. It seems like there is no liquid at first, but just hang in there; it gets really juicy.

Let cool and serve on anything!

CHERRY TOMATO CHUTNEY

MAKES ABOUT 2½ CUPS

The Healthy Librarian, Debbie Kastner, eats plant-based and posts the most current evidence-based research on plant-based food on her blog. She got us hooked on this after she shared a fantastic recipe using this chutney as a pizza topping. It is beautiful and delicious. The inspiration for the chutney came from Bobby Flay, though we have tweaked it to be more plant perfect. This is the beautiful topping on the Tomato Chutney over Caramelized Onion Hummus Pizza (page 198).

INGREDIENTS:

- ½ yellow onion, thinly sliced
- 3 cloves garlic, minced
- 2 pints grape or cherry tomatoes
- ¼ cup apple cider vinegar
- 1 tablespoon maple syrup
- Pinch of ground allspice
- Pinch of ground cinnamon
- Pinch of freshly ground black pepper
- 2 tablespoons chopped fresh cilantro (optional)

INSTRUCTIONS:

In a medium saucepan, cook the onions over high heat, stirring, until they brown slightly. Reduce the heat in increments as the onions continue to soften, brown, and caramelize. Add small amounts of water if the onions get dry or start to stick to the pan. The water will deglaze the pan.

Add the garlic, and cook for just 30 seconds. Add the tomatoes (do not cut them!), ¼ cup water, the vinegar, maple syrup, allspice, cinnamon, and pepper. Cook until the tomatoes soften and the mixture thickens, 20 minutes or a tad longer.

The dish is so beautiful at this stage—it is almost a shame to do anything more! Remove from the heat when the excess liquid is completely absorbed and stir in the cilantro. Let cool to room temperature.

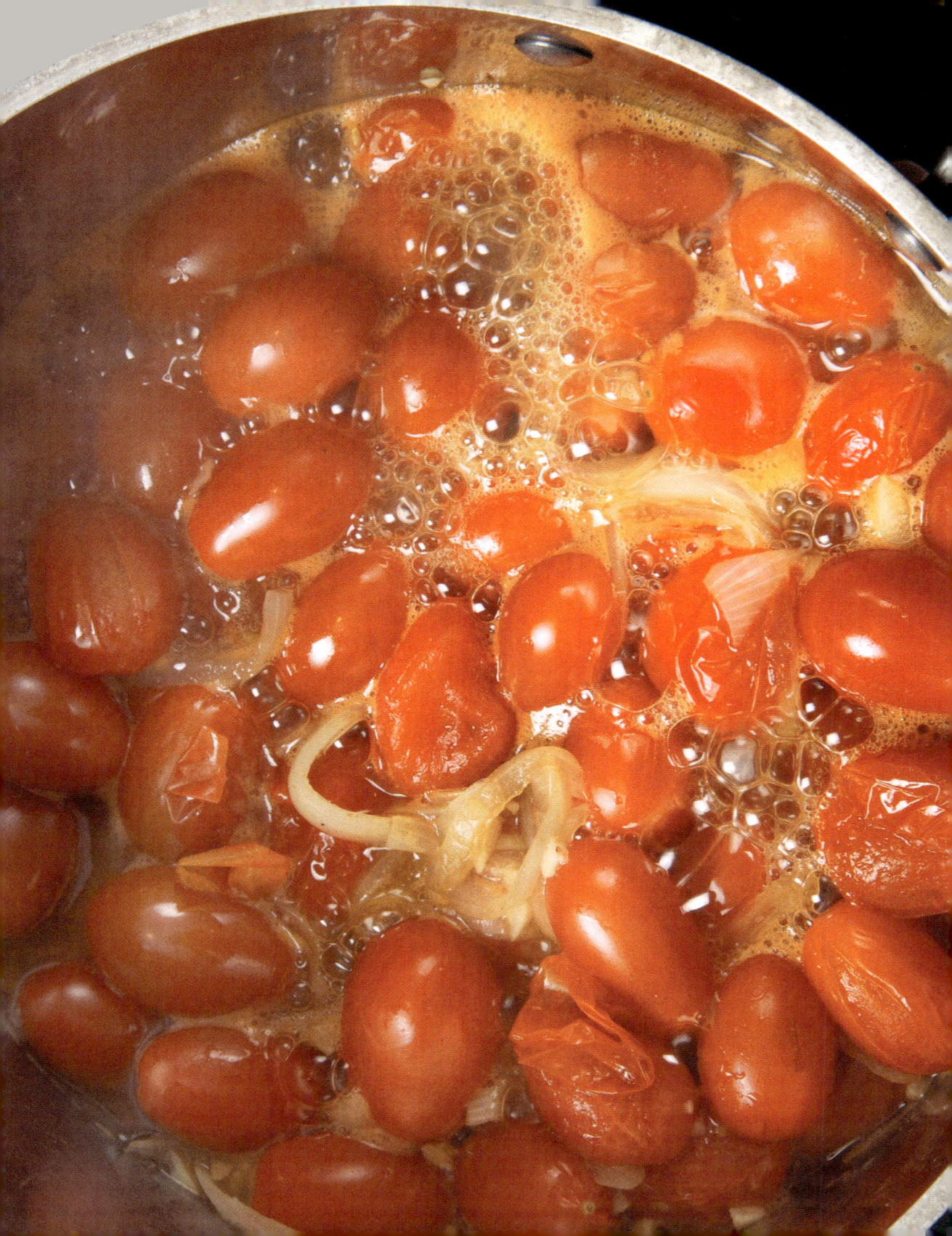

CANNELLINI BEAN SAUCE

This was the answer to our prayers. We needed to make a nut-free version of our favorite sauce, the OMG Walnut Sauce from My Beef with Meat, *to use on greens, as a base for dressings, and, most important, on our favorite appetizer, Kale Bruschetta (page 60). The cover has a photo of "Enlightened" Dr. Seuss Stacked Polenta (page 130) with this sauce.*

INGREDIENTS:

  1 (15-ounce) can no-salt-added cannellini beans, drained and rinsed

  1 to 2 cloves garlic

  2 tablespoons low-sodium tamari

INSTRUCTIONS:

In a food processor, combine the beans, garlic, and tamari, and process until very smooth, adding water as needed until the desired texture is reached; use more water for a thinner dressing, less water for a thicker dip. Serve over kale, greens, salads, grains, or veggies, or use as a spread for sandwiches or as a topping on pizza.

SWEET CORN SAUCE

This sauce is easy and quick to make and looks pretty sprinkled with parsley, cilantro, or dill. Use it on top of greens or grains or try it on our favorite Asparagus Mushroom Pie (page 202). It is so delicious you might even like it alone by the spoonful! It is best made with fresh corn. If you use frozen corn be sure it tastes sweet, and thaw under running water first.

INGREDIENTS:

5 ears fresh corn, or 16 ounces frozen sweet corn, thawed

1 cup chopped sweet onion

½ to 1 cup low-sodium vegetable stock or water

1 tablespoon balsamic vinegar (white balsamic keeps the sauce light in color)

INSTRUCTIONS:

If using fresh corn, cut the kernels off the corn cobs and scrape the cobs to extract any juice. Place the corn in a blender along with the onions and ½ cup of the stock and puree.

Put blended mixture in a pan and cook like scrambled eggs, stirring until it is warmed through and just starting to bubble. Add more stock if necessary. A thinner sauce is better over greens. Add balsamic vinegar and stir again. This also makes a good salad dressing with more vinegar, lemon juice, or lime juice to taste.

LEMONY CHEEZY SAUCE

There is no cheese substitute in the Prevent and Reverse Heart Disease program, but this looks like cheese and has the "meltiness" factor of cheese, too. Turmeric makes it a wonderful cheesy yellow color, and red pepper hummus (we recommend Engine 2 brand) enhances the flavor even more. For a thicker sauce, use an extra tablespoon of cornstarch. Then it is really cheesy! We love it on homemade pita chips, with vegetables, over cauliflower, or melted under the broiler on English muffins with tomatoes and greens—and actually, sometimes we like it just by the spoonful. It is the deliciousness in the Asparagus Mushroom Pie with Lemony Cheezy Sauce (page 202). Crazily, this sauce looks like Hollandaise. Fortunately, it is not!

INGREDIENTS:

½ cup nutritional yeast

½ cup Our Hummus (page 102) or hummus prepared without oil or tahini

¾ cup low-sodium vegetable broth or water

¼ teaspoon ground turmeric

Pinch of cayenne pepper

1 tablespoon cornstarch

Zest of ½ lemon

2 to 3 tablespoons fresh lemon juice, to taste

INSTRUCTIONS:

In a saucepan, combine the nutritional yeast, hummus, broth, turmeric, cayenne, cornstarch, and lemon zest and juice over medium heat, stirring continuously with a wire whisk, until the sauce thickens. Remove from the heat when it just starts to boil—it will be nice and thick and ready to use!

RASPBERRY SAUCE

We are crazy about this sauce on almost anything: waffles, pancakes, cut-up fruit, or even toast! It is better than maple syrup. Try it on toasted Engine 2 brown rice tortillas—awesome! In this recipe, the vinegar adds a little zing. If you make it in smaller amounts, use about ½ teaspoon balsamic vinegar to ½ cup raspberries. This sauce is especially good using raspberry balsamic vinegar!

INGREDIENTS:

   10 ounces frozen raspberries, thawed

   1 teaspoon balsamic vinegar, or more to taste

INSTRUCTIONS:

In a food processor, combine the raspberries and vinegar, and process until uniformly smooth. Use immediately or refrigerate until ready to use.

ENCHILADA SAUCE

This sauce gives flavor and kick to the Tortilla Azteca (page 196) and many other Mexican-inspired dishes. Make a batch and store it in the fridge. It adds a nice depth of flavor to food. Try it on the Shrapnel Burrito (page 214), Breakfast Hash (page 51), or Chile Rellenos (page 218).

INGREDIENTS:

2 tablespoons whole wheat flour

¼ cup chili powder

½ teaspoon garlic powder

½ teaspoon onion powder

½ teaspoon ground cumin

¼ teaspoon dried oregano

2 cups low-sodium vegetable broth

6 ounces tomato paste

¼ teaspoon salt (optional)

INSTRUCTIONS:

In a small bowl, combine the flour, chili powder, garlic powder, onion powder, cumin, and oregano, and stir.

In a saucepan over medium heat, combine the broth, the small bowl of flour and spice mixture, the tomato paste, and salt (if using). Stir well to combine and dissolve the tomato paste. Simmer over low heat for at least 20 minutes, stirring occasionally. Add more spices as desired.

SHIITAKE MUSHROOM AND ONION GRAVY

There is just nothing like the flavor and texture of shiitake mushrooms. It is tempting to cover everything with this gravy, but we love it most of all on the Good Garlicky Mashed Potatoes (page 138). Try it anywhere you choose: on toast, pasta, rice, vegetables! That's what Essy does— anywhere and everywhere!

INGREDIENTS:

- 1 large sweet onion, chopped
- 2 cups sliced shiitake mushrooms
- 4 cups vegetable broth
- ⅓ cup whole wheat, rice, spelt, or any whole-grain flour
- ¼ teaspoon dried sage, crumbled
- ¼ teaspoon dried thyme
- ¼ teaspoon freshly ground black pepper
- 1 to 2 tablespoons low-sodium tamari (optional)

INSTRUCTIONS:

In a large frying pan, cook the onions over medium heat until they start to become translucent. Add the shiitakes, cover, and cook, stirring occasionally, for about 10 minutes, until soft.

Add the broth, and continue cooking until heated through.

Add the flour, stirring with a whisk to avoid lumps, and cook, stirring occasionally, for 10 minutes.

Add the sage, thyme, and pepper, and you are ready to serve this on anything! Taste and add a tablespoon or two of tamari if absolutely necessary. We find this just fabulous as it is, without the tamari!

MOMMY'S MUSHROOM GRAVY 2.0

This gravy is too good! At Thanksgiving, it is the first dish empty on the buffet. It is similar to the recipe in My Beef with Meat; *however, we trimmed down the amount of tamari and miso to lower the sodium content. And we offer a gluten-free flour mixture option, for those with gluten allergies. This is the gravy used in the Roasted Red New Potatoes and Gravy recipe (page 140). Also try it on top of Good Garlicky Mashed Potatoes (page 138) and with Brian's Stuffing (page 136).*

INGREDIENTS:

1 onion, chopped

2 to 3 cloves garlic, minced

12 ounces mushrooms, sliced

2 cups vegetable broth

2 teaspoons white miso (white has the lowest sodium content)

2 tablespoons gluten-free flour mixture or whole wheat flour

2 tablespoons low-sodium tamari

2 tablespoons cooking sherry (optional)

Freshly ground black pepper

INSTRUCTIONS:

In a saucepan, cook the onions over medium-high heat, stirring and adding a splash of water to the pan if they start to burn. Allow the onions to brown a little. Add the garlic and mushrooms, and continue cooking until the mushrooms soften. Again, add a splash of water, as needed, to keep the mixture from burning.

Add 1 cup of the broth to the pan, and stir.

To the remaining cup of broth, add the miso, flour, and tamari, and stir until dissolved. Add the dissolved miso and flour mixture to the pan along with the sherry (if using). Continue cooking until the gravy thickens to your liking. Season with pepper to taste. Serve warm.

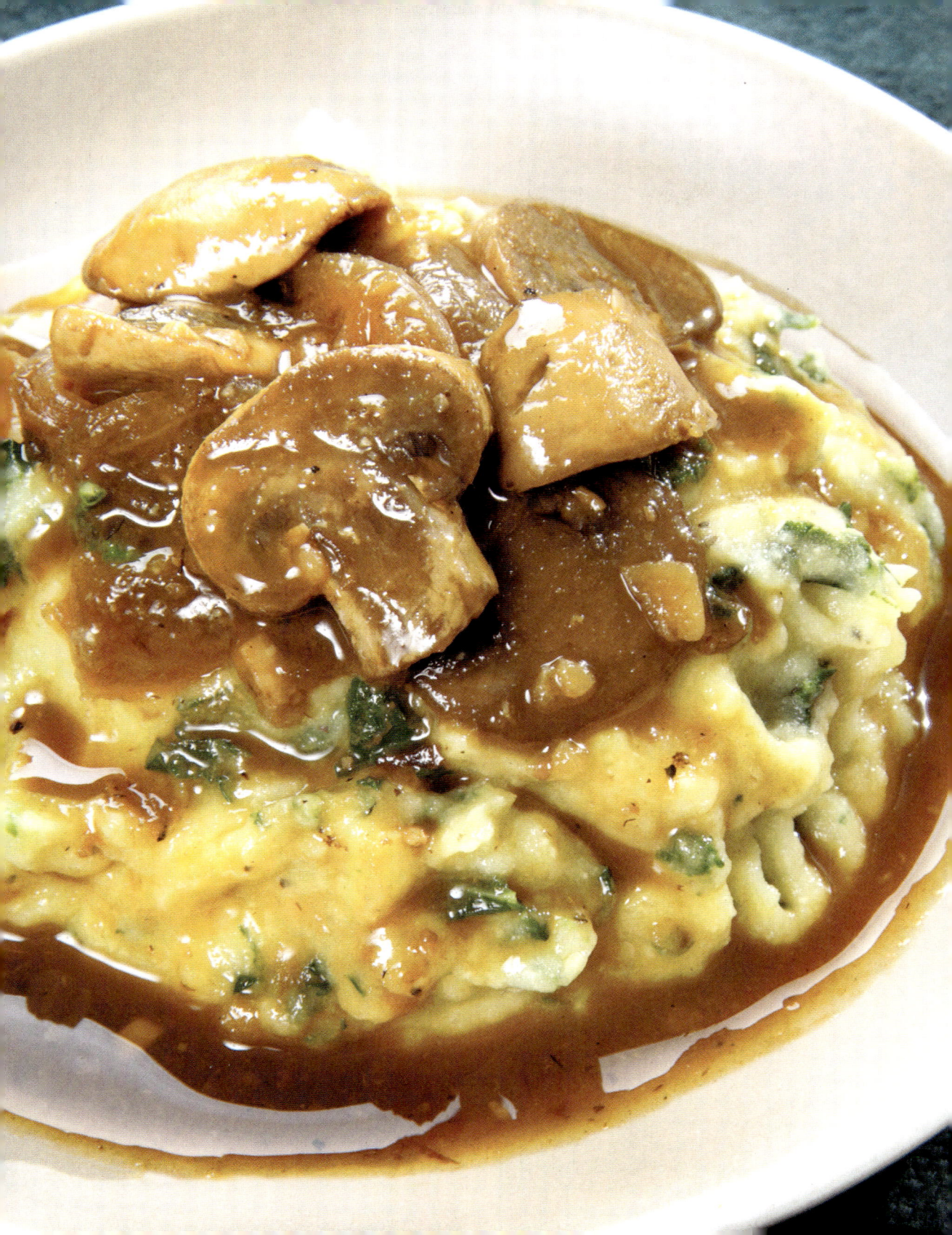

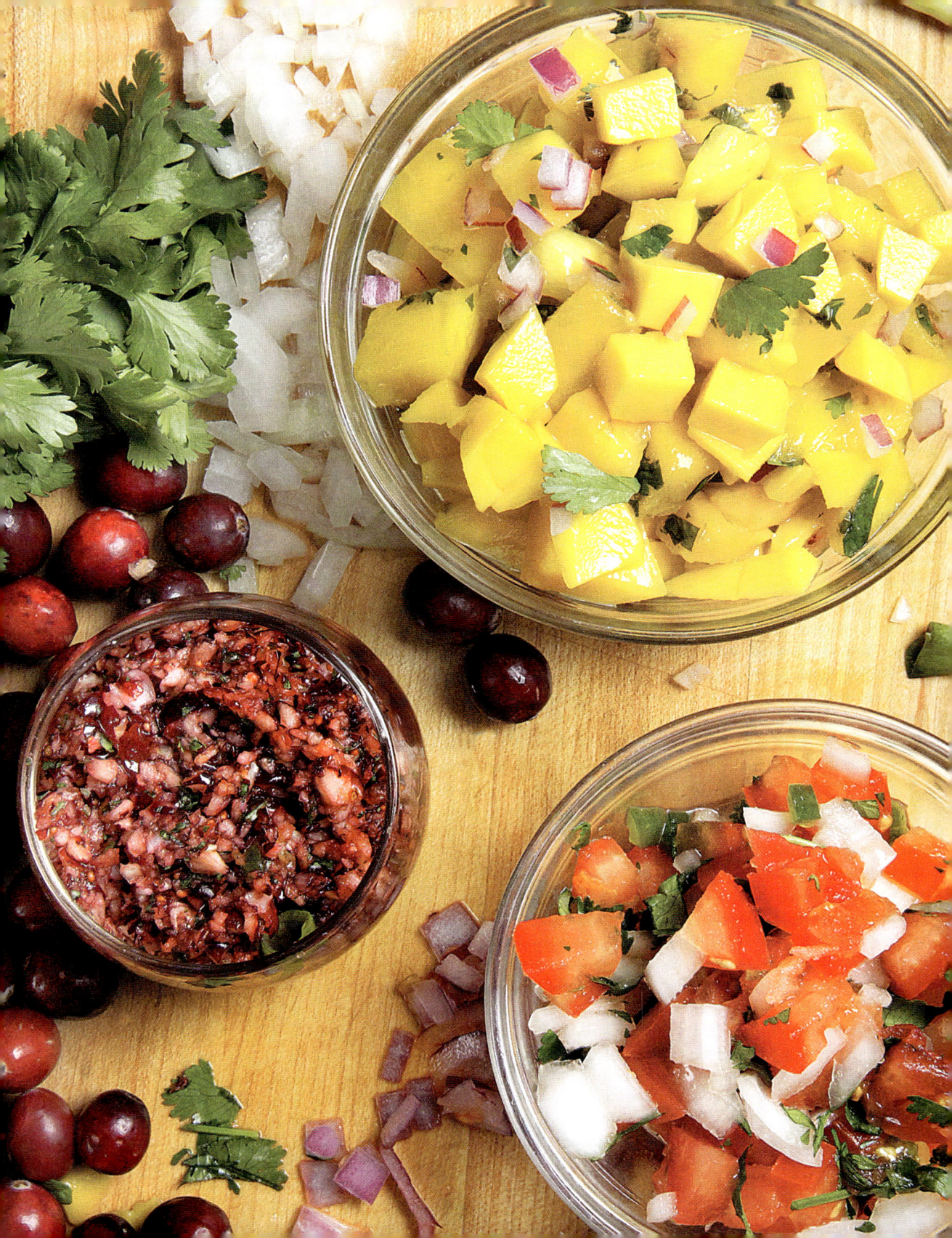

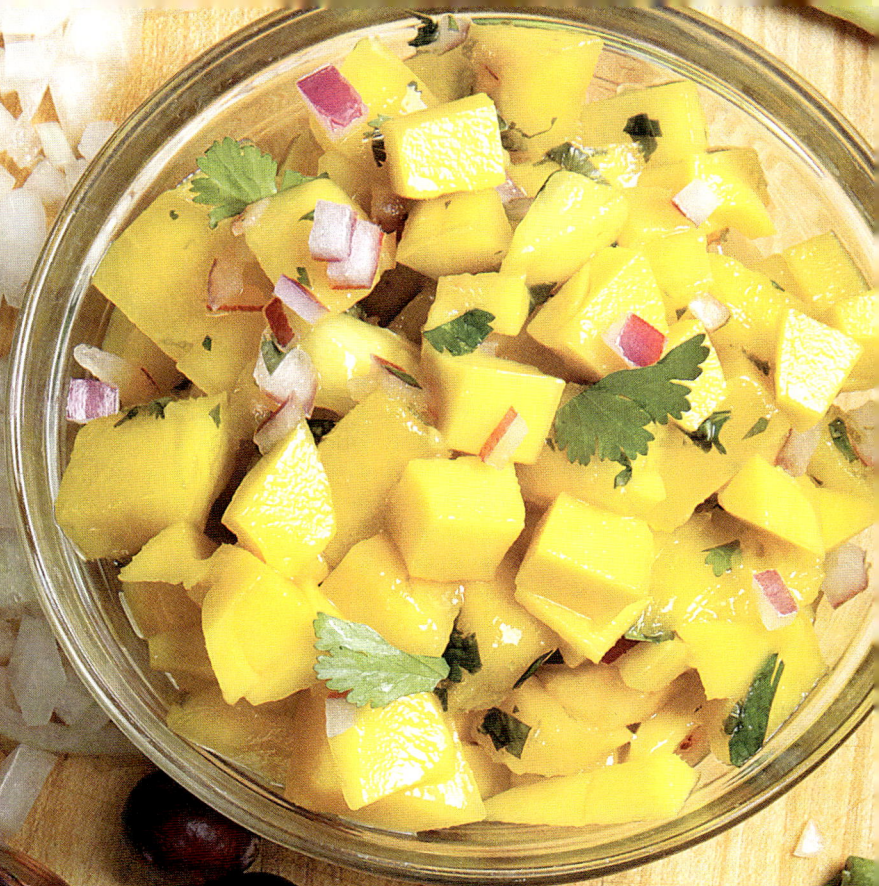

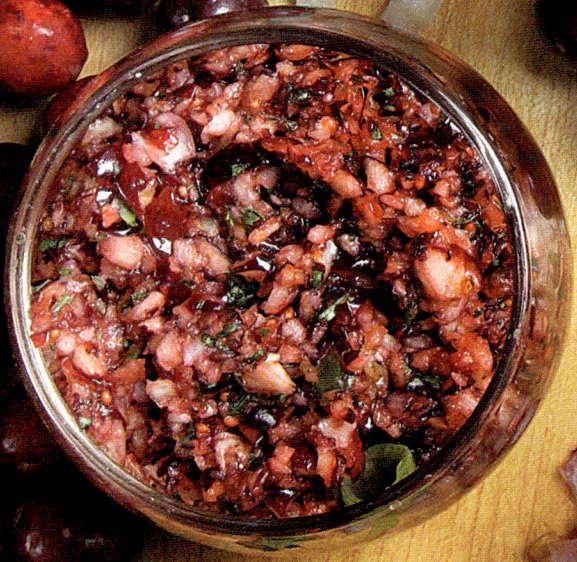

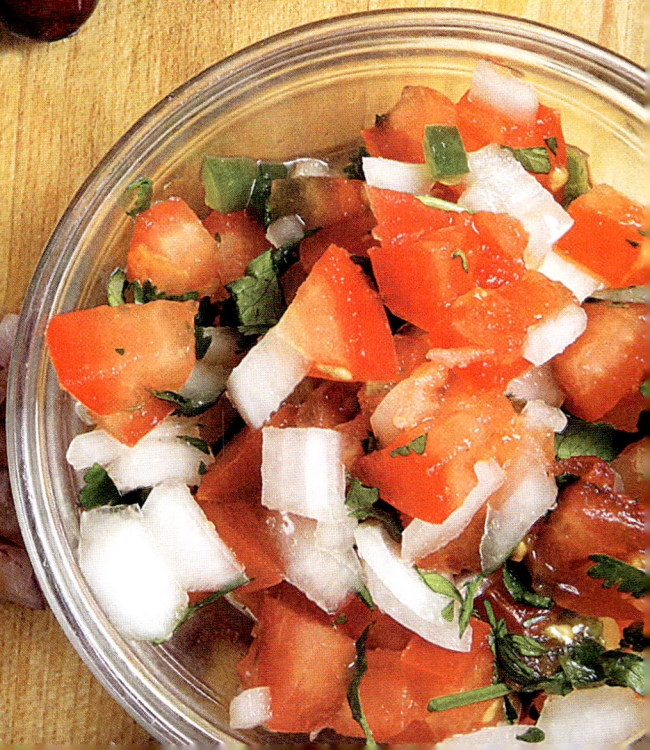

Salsas: It is all about the toppings.

Salsas are usually made without oil, yet they sometimes have unnecessarily high amounts of sodium. We have created some really delicious salsas that transform anything you are eating into wonderful explosions of taste, color, and flavor!

Do not miss out on the fun of making these. Some may be seasonal for where you live, so keep your eyes open for what will make great fresh salsas for you!

PICO DE GALLO

MAKES 2 CUPS

In Spanish, pico de gallo means "rooster's beak." There is no rooster in this dish at all—it is a fresh, simple, nutritionally dense, delicious display of Mother Nature at her best. We like to combine this with other salsas. It is not too hot and not too sweet—so pair it with the flavor you seek. We serve it alongside the Shrapnel Burrito (page 214), Black Bean and Sweet Potato–Collard Burrito (page 212), Five-Star Rice and Beans (page 208), Matt's Sofrito Black Beans (page 211), or anywhere!

INGREDIENTS:

2 cups tomatoes, cored and diced

¼ cup white onion, diced

½ jalapeño, seeded and diced

1 tablespoon minced garlic

Juice of 2 lemons

¼ cup fresh cilantro, finely chopped

INSTRUCTIONS:

In a bowl, combine the tomatoes, onion, jalapeño, garlic, lemon juice, and cilantro. Stir and serve immediately, or cover and chill until ready to serve.

MANGO-LIME SALSA

I could eat this salsa every single day. Its flavors are so bright that it always gives me a lift. The other night at dinner my dad said, "You could put this Mango-Lime Salsa on a slate shingle and it would taste good." We love this on Matt's Sofrito Black Beans (page 209) and one hundred thousand other things!

INGREDIENTS:

2 ripe mangoes, pitted, peeled, and diced

¼ red onion, minced

½ cup chopped fresh parsley or cilantro

Zest of 1 lime

Juice of 1½ limes

INSTRUCTIONS:

In a bowl, combine the mango, onion, parsley, lime zest, and lime juice, and mix. Serve over anything that needs a lift!

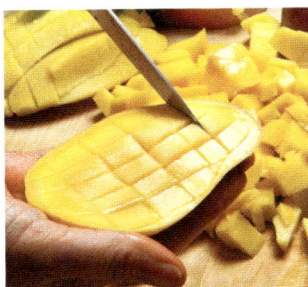

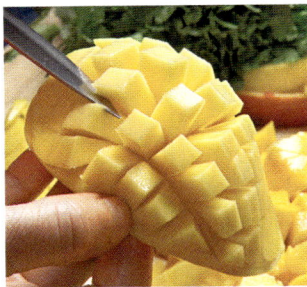

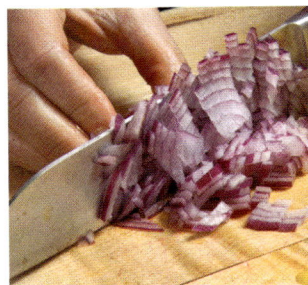

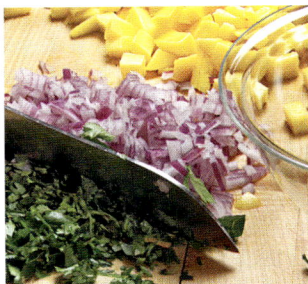

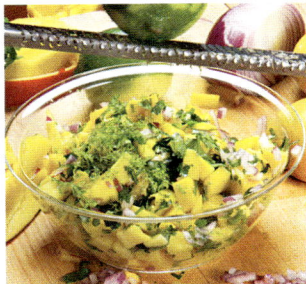

DOWN UNDER CRANBERRY SALSA

How ironic that an Australian pal passed along the recipe for this salsa—they don't even grow cranberries down under! But thanks to that friend, Leanne, for sharing this unique family recipe. It is now one of our favorite salsas and we use it on almost everything. Try it with Brian's Stuffing (page 136), with toasted whole wheat pita, on top of Five-Star Rice and Beans (page 206), or with anything that needs zip. Seriously, we eat this year-round. It works with fresh or frozen cranberries, so no worries, mate. Go for it, even down under!

INGREDIENTS:

- 1 (12-ounce) package fresh or frozen cranberries
- 3 tablespoons fresh lime juice
- ½ to ¾ cup pure maple syrup
- 3 to 4 green onions, thinly sliced
- ½ large jalapeño, seeded and chopped
- 2 cups fresh cilantro leaves, not chopped

INSTRUCTIONS:

Place the cranberries, lime juice, maple syrup, green onions, jalapeño, and cilantro in a food processor, and process just until coarsely chopped. Chill and serve.

TIP:

Blending the mixture longer turns this salsa into more of a relish, which can be delish!

ROASTED TOMATILLO SALSA

When you roast the ingredients in this recipe it completely transforms them. The resulting flavors are mild, amazing, even buttery. This salsa thrills us.

INGREDIENTS:

4 tomatillos, husked, rinsed well, and dried

¼ large onion

1 long, skinny green chile (also called a finger chile)

1 large clove garlic

About ¼ cup fresh cilantro

INSTRUCTIONS:

Roast the tomatillos, onion, chile, and garlic over a gas flame or even on the stovetop of an electric stove, if you are bold. Once the ingredients blacken in different areas, they are ready.

Or, if you prefer, preheat the broiler. Place the tomatillos, onion, chile, and garlic on a foil-lined baking sheet and broil them, watching carefully in case they begin to burn too much. Once the vegetables begin to blacken in different areas, they are ready. Set aside to cool.

Once cooled, remove the seeds from the chile pepper if you desire less heat. Leave some seeds in for more heat. It is up to you.

Place the roasted tomatillos, onion, chile, garlic, and cilantro in the food processor, and process until it reaches the salsa texture you desire. Serve.

SHOW-OFF PEACH SALSA

When peaches are in season and at their peak deliciousness, I buy twenty at a time. If we don't get through them all before the fruit flies invade, I use the softer ones, the ones the kids pass over, to make the magic of this delicious peach salsa. It is out of this world. I feel like a show-off even though it's all due to the peaches, not me!

INGREDIENTS:

- 2 peaches, just past ripe, peeled and cubed (about 2 cups)
- 2 green onions, chopped
- 2 cloves garlic, finely minced
- 2 cups diced tomatoes
- 2 tablespoons minced parsley
- Shake or two of hot sauce, your choice (optional)

INSTRUCTIONS:

Combine the peaches, green onions, garlic, tomatoes, parsley, and hot sauce, if using, in a bowl. Stir together, serve, and get ready to be called a "show-off"!

POMEGRANATE SALSA

This is a delicious, vibrant salsa that has no added sweetener other than the pomegranates. It is convenient but expensive to buy the pomegranates already prepared. However, it is also fun to remove the seeds yourself and especially easy to do if you put the pomegranate in a bowl of water in the sink. What's so cool is that the seeds sink and the white pith floats! This salsa enhances anything from the most simple dish to the most complex . . . from toast to beans and rice to anything else that needs a boost of flavor.

INGREDIENTS:

 1 cup pomegranate seeds

 Zest of 1 lime

 2 tablespoons fresh lime juice

 2 green onions, white and green parts finely chopped

INSTRUCTIONS:

Combine the pomegranate seeds, lime zest, lime juice, and green onions in a small bowl. Stir and serve. You will be the talk of the town!

There are only a few commercially sold pasta sauces available without oil. Know that now, so you don't waste a lot of time reading the labels on all of them. Nothing is more frustrating than standing forever in front of the pasta sauces in the grocery store looking at all the listed ingredients, especially when more often than not there isn't one on the shelf made without oil. And you have been standing there forever.

Look primarily for Walnut Acres organic low-sodium tomato sauce if you can find it. We've found a handful of other sauces with no added oil, but this one is the best. You may find others available near you, but remember the ingredient label is key. It is wonderful to have a supply of good pasta sauces on hand in a pinch. But in this section, we'll give you some fast and easy tomato sauce recipes you can make yourself with no added oil or salt. We've also included some delicious and hearty taco and enchilada sauces here.

The truth is, nothing in the grocery store is equal to the recipes Jane has created!

LIGHT AND EASY MARINARA

MAKES 7 CUPS

There are so many ways to make your own marinara by adding different spices or veggies. This one is my favorite because there is no chopping or prep needed. This light and easy recipe is fantastic alone (or you may add your favorite veggies, if you have the inclination!). Cook this a bit longer and the sauce gets darker and thicker—which can be great if you want to use it as a pizza sauce.

INGREDIENTS:

- 1 (28-ounce) can diced tomatoes
- 1 (28-ounce) can crushed tomatoes
- 2 teaspoons dried thyme
- 2 teaspoons dried rosemary
- 2 teaspoons dried oregano
- 1 teaspoon onion powder
- 1 teaspoon minced garlic
- 2 to 3 tablespoons maple syrup

INSTRUCTIONS:

In a medium saucepan, combine the diced tomatoes, crushed tomatoes, thyme, rosemary, oregano, onion powder, garlic, and maple syrup. Simmer over medium-high heat for 5 minutes. Reduce the heat to low and simmer until ready to serve.

BESTO PESTO

Pesto is just the besto. This is a rich bean-based pesto sauce without all that oil and cheese. There are all sorts of plant-based recipes out there for similar pestos, but our recipe highlights my mom's love of lemon juice and lemon zest.

INGREDIENTS:

1 (15-ounce) can cannellini beans, drained and rinsed

2 cloves garlic, chopped

¼ cup nutritional yeast

Zest of ½ lemon, or more as desired

¼ cup fresh lemon juice, or more as desired

1 cup packed fresh basil

INSTRUCTIONS:

In a food processor, combine the beans, garlic, nutritional yeast, lemon zest, lemon juice, and basil, and process until smooth.

Serve over pasta, as a spread, as a dip, or as a dressing.

BASIL AND LEEK MARINARA

Most tomato products need some sugar to cut the acid, but here the balsamic vinegar does the trick! Use this pasta sauce anywhere you need a great-tasting sauce. My husband is a sauce man, and I can say only that there is almost nothing that has not been anointed with Basil and Leek Marinara!

INGREDIENTS:

    1 large onion, chopped

    1 leek (white and light green parts), chopped

    4 cloves garlic, chopped

    1 (28-ounce) can, no-salt whole peeled tomatoes (Cento San Marzano brand
        recommended)

    Pinch of red pepper flakes

    1 cup fresh basil, chopped, or 1 tablespoon dried

    1 tablespoon balsamic vinegar, or to taste

    ½ teaspoon black pepper

INSTRUCTIONS:

Place onions, leeks, and garlic in a large pan, and cook over medium heat, stirring occasionally, and adding drops of water or broth as necessary if the pan gets dry. Cook until the onions and leeks are reduced, translucent, and very soft.

Add tomatoes, red pepper flakes, and basil to the onions and leeks. Put your hands in the pot and squeeze each tomato until it loses its shape. Careful: They squirt. It's fun! Stir, cover, and cook on low heat for 15 more minutes.

With an immersion blender right in the pot or in a food processor, blend the sauce a little bit. Our thirteen-year-old grandson thinks it should be smooth, and we like having a few chunks—but it is your call how much you want to blend or not.

Add balsamic vinegar and pepper, stir, and serve over pasta or anything that needs a sauce.

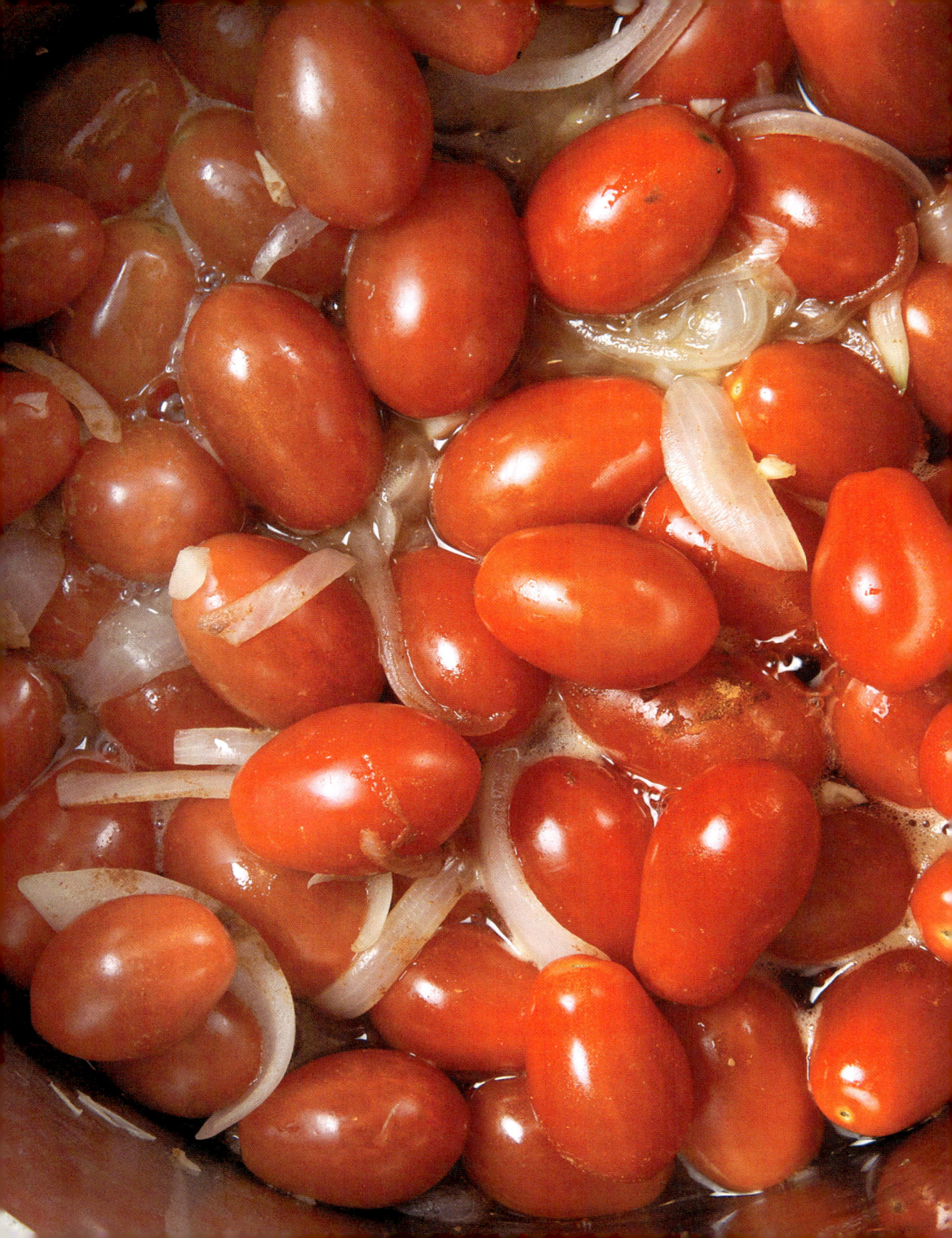

APPETIZERS AND SIDES

Vegetables—the whole rainbow of vegetables—should fill your plate every day. Aim for all the colors and then always throw in leafy greens any way you can, cooked or not, at every meal.

How long or even whether you cook your greens is up to you. We like cooked kale, collards, Swiss chard, etc., and feel that when you cook these greens, it's a good way to eat more of them. Our favorite thing to put on greens is a wonderful balsamic vinegar. As my husband says, "A sprinkle of balsamic vinegar changes kale and collards to a hot fudge sundae!"

Asparagus, broccoli, green beans, cauliflower, and peas are quick to cook and wonderful with any meal. And experiment with less familiar vegetables, too. Artichokes are a favorite of ours to linger over with special guests. Beets, colorful and red or pale pink Chioggia, brighten any plate. Brussels sprouts are wonderful dipped in hummus or even broiled. Potatoes, sweet and white, are filling and can be made in endless variations.

We were fortunate to be given a French-fry cutter, which we have mounted on the kitchen wall. In a flash we can make white or sweet potato fries by pressing a potato through the cutter and baking the fries in the oven on parchment paper.

Leftover vegetables are great in salads or just for a quick snack, though sadly, we rarely have leftovers in the vegetable category! It is crazy how easy it is to eat whole plates full of asparagus or broccoli when they are cooked just the way we like—beginning to be soft but not at all mushy! Everyone has his or her own taste, from crisp to mush. Eat what you love, and if it is vegetables—FEAST!

Some of these recipes can be stand-alone dinners, too. Jane and our editor don't understand my insistence that mashed potatoes should be the center of the meal so they are here, against my will, in this section. But if you wish, treat them or anything you choose as the main event and build your meal around them.

"ENLIGHTENED" DR. SEUSS STACKED POLENTA

This recipe received more acclaim than any other (except for the Adonis Cake) in My Beef with Meat. *The comments included: "This is a* perfect *food!," "This is my favorite thing I have ever eaten," "We are serving this at our wedding—it is so elegant." The small amount of OMG Walnut Sauce in the original is the only part of the recipe that is not plant-perfect. So, we have created a new* enlightened *version of this favorite dish with a plant-perfect Cannellini Bean Sauce (page 110)!*

INGREDIENTS

1 sweet potato, roughly the same girth as the polenta

1 tube precooked polenta

3 to 4 tomatoes, roughly the same girth as the polenta

1 bunch cilantro or basil, your preference, leaves only

1 lime or lemon, your preference

1 cup Cannellini Bean Sauce (page 110)

1 bottle balsamic glaze (we recommend Isola Classic Cream of Balsamic, which is deceptively named as there is no cream in it!)

INSTRUCTIONS:

Preheat the oven to 350°F. Line two baking sheets with parchment paper.

Slice the sweet potato into ⅓-inch-thick rounds.

Place the sweet potato rounds on one of the lined baking sheets and bake for 30 to 40 minutes, or until cooked through. Count the number of sweet potato rounds you have created.

Slice the tube of polenta into ⅓-inch-thick rounds, making sure you have the same number of sweet potatoes rounds.

Place the polenta slices on the other lined baking sheet and bake for 20 minutes, until they are warmed through.

Slice the tomatoes in thick, round slices—again making sure you have the same number of slices as the polenta and sweet potato rounds.

To make the cilantro-lime topping or basil-lemon topping, combine the cilantro with the juice of 1 lime in a small food processor and pulse until coarsely chopped, or combine the basil with the juice of 1 lemon and pulse until coarsely chopped.

Place the polenta rounds on a handsome serving platter. Spread a layer of Cannellini Bean Sauce on top of each polenta round. Stack one sweet potato round on top of each sauce-coated polenta round. Spread a layer of sauce on top of each sweet potato round. Place a tomato slice on top of the sweet potato layer.

Dollop the cilantro-lime topping or basil-lemon topping on top of the tomato layer. Drizzle the top and sides of the stacks as well as the plate with the balsamic glaze in a star pattern.

Serve with a sharp knife and fork. Rave on!

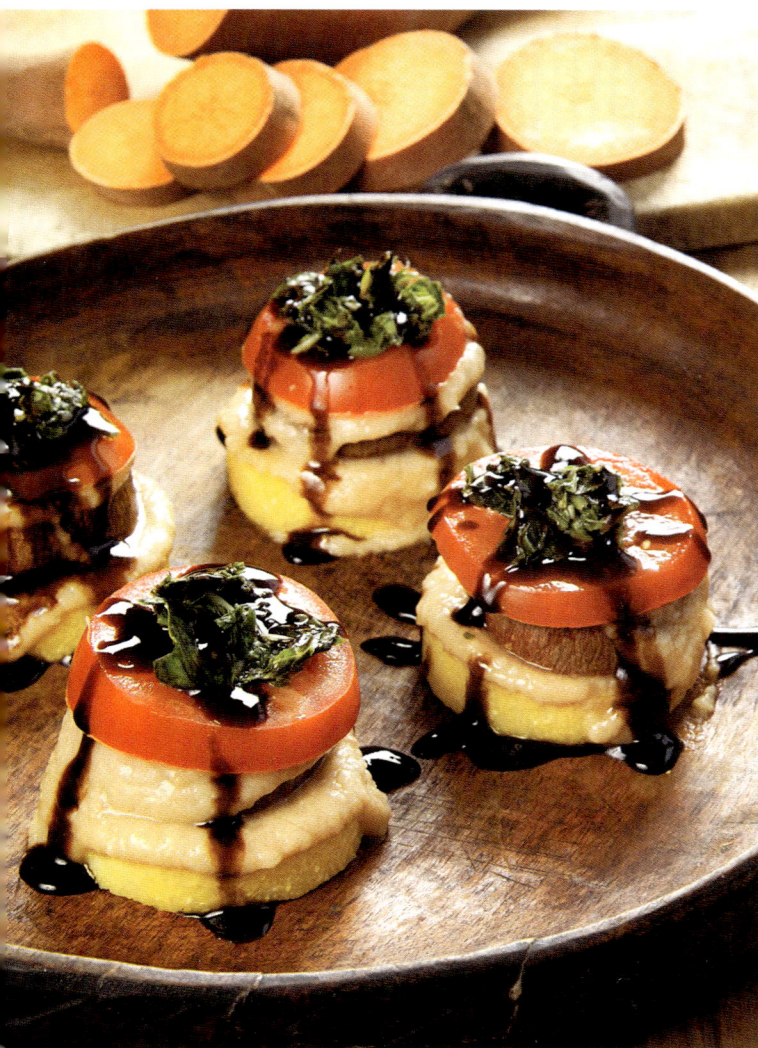

SMOKY LITTLE DEVILS

These tiny stuffed potatoes are absolutely beautiful, and, oh so delicious as hors d'oeuvres or the center part of a meal. Be sure the potatoes are tiny. And remember to hold back! Don't eat them all before your guests arrive!

INGREDIENTS:

12 small red potatoes (roughly the size of large walnuts or small clementines)

1⅓ cups Green Onion Hummus (page 103)

Pinch of smoked paprika, for garnish

1 green onion, finely sliced, for garnish

Baby kale leaves, for garnish (optional)

INSTRUCTIONS:

Set a steamer insert in a saucepan and add about 2 inches of water. Bring to a boil over high heat; then place the potatoes in the steamer basket and steam for about 20 minutes. Plunge them into cold water in a big bowl or just run cold water over them.

Slice each potato in half. With the small end of a melon-baller or a small spoon, scoop out a hole in the center. (Save the little scooped-out potato balls to put into a salad or just pop them into your mouth!)

Fill each hole with Green Onion Hummus. Sprinkle with smoked paprika. It is easiest to take a tiny bit between your fingers and sprinkle just enough for the color to show.

Garnish with green onions or, for a really fun look, use a tiny baby kale leaf as a "sail" in each little potato "boat."

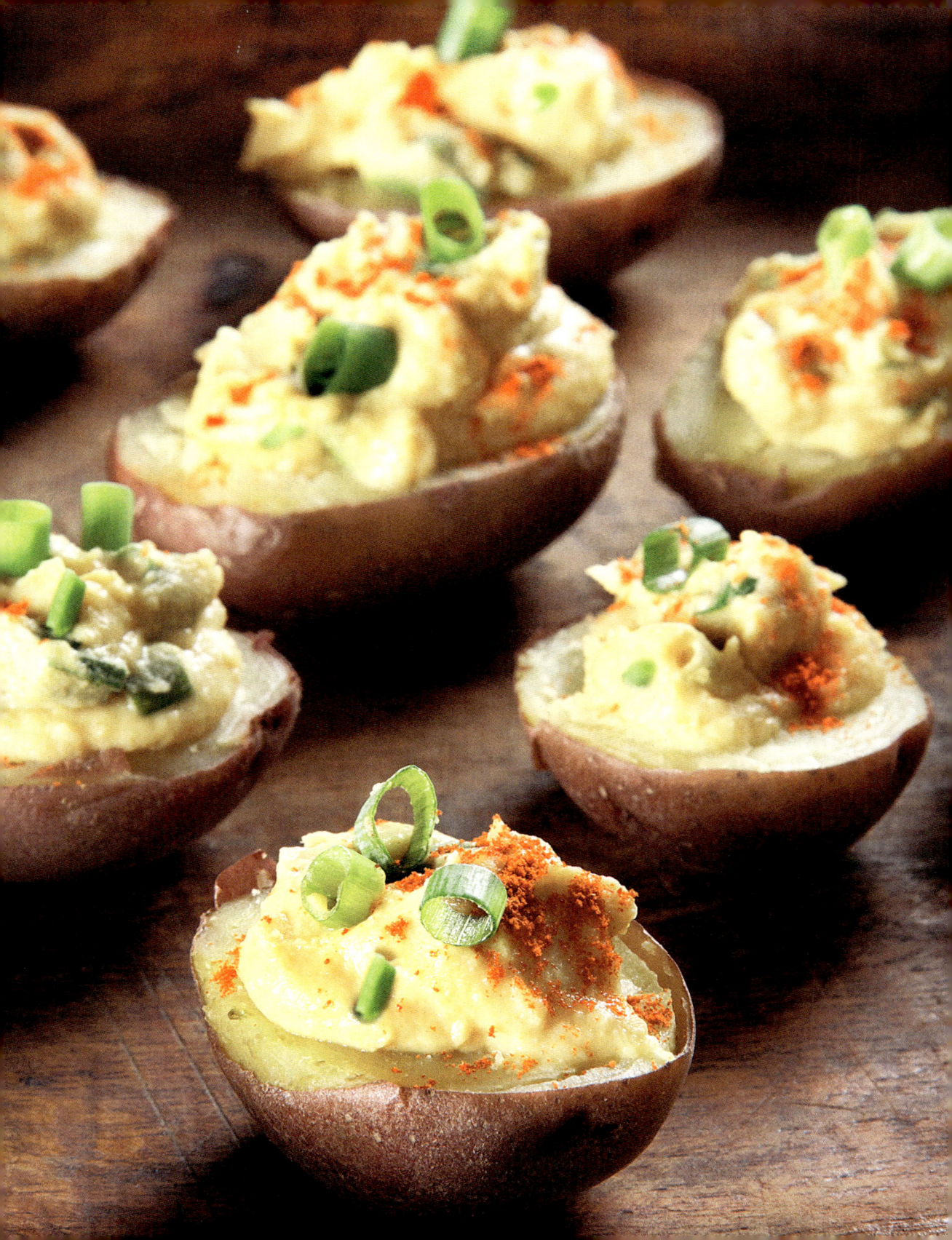

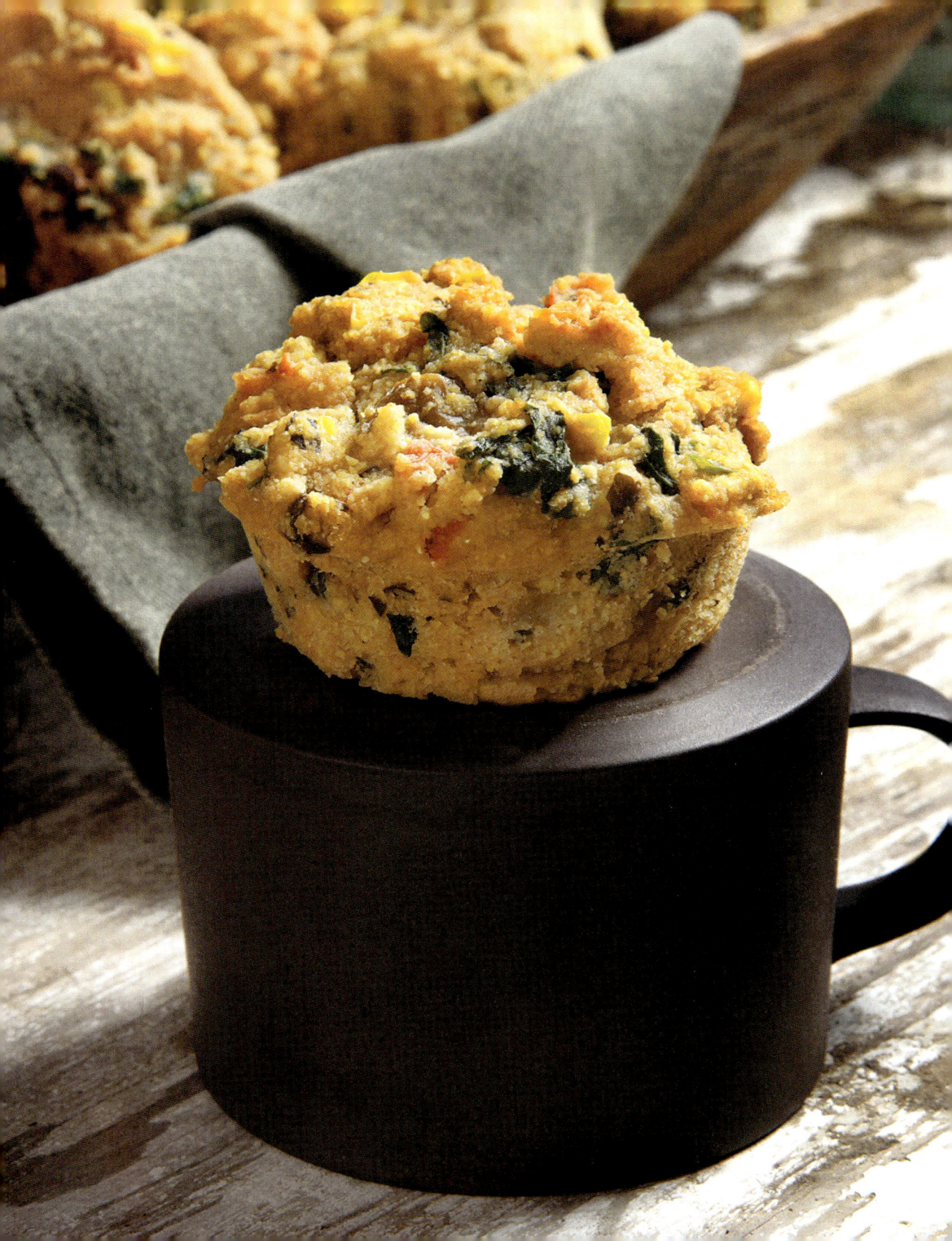

JALAPEÑO AND SALSA CORN MUFFINS

These savory muffins have been wowing crowds across the country. We serve them at breakfast in our Engine 2 Retreats and see many people squirreling them away for a mid-morning snack!

INGREDIENTS:

1 cup diced onion

1 jalapeño, seeded and chopped

2 cups kale, stems removed and leaves chopped into bite-size pieces

¾ cup fresh or frozen corn

1 cup cornmeal

1 cup white whole wheat flour or oat flour

1 teaspoon baking soda

½ cup unsweetened oat milk

¼ cup unsweetened applesauce

3 tablespoons pure maple syrup

1 cup salsa

INSTRUCTIONS:

Preheat the oven to 400°F.

In a frying pan, cook the onion, jalapeño, kale, and corn over medium-high heat for 5 minutes, or until all the vegetables are cooked through. Add a teaspoon or two of water if the pan gets dry. Set aside.

In a large bowl, combine the cornmeal, flour, and baking soda. Add the oat milk, applesauce, and maple syrup, and stir to combine. Add the cooked veggies and the salsa, and stir the batter until well mixed.

Divide the batter evenly among the wells of a standard muffin tin. Bake for 25 to 28 minutes. Eat while they are hot!

BRIAN'S STUFFING

My husband, Brian, makes this stuffing at Thanksgiving. My mom loves it so much she asks for it for Christmas. Sure enough, her gift from Brian each year is a big pan of his stuffing, and we feast on it for Christmas Day lunch! Here's a fun twist: Cook and serve this stuffing inside a pumpkin. Seriously! Find a cooking pumpkin that will fit inside your oven, clean out the insides, stuff the open space with stuffing, place the lid back on, and cook as described below. We love this with Down Under Cranberry Salsa (page 121) and Mommy's Mushroom Gravy 2.0 (page 116). You will, too!

INGREDIENTS:

15 pieces of bread with no added oil: 5 multigrain, 5 dark rye, and 5 whole wheat, cut into 1-inch cubes

1 large onion, diced

3 cups chopped celery

1 cup kale, stems stripped and leaves chopped into bite-size pieces

2 cups slivered carrots

16 ounces mushrooms, sliced

4 ounces water chestnuts, sliced

2 apples, cored and diced

1 pear, cored and diced

2 tablespoons dried sage, crumbled

2 teaspoon dried thyme

1 tablespoon dried oregano

1 teaspoon garlic powder

½ teaspoon freshly ground black pepper

4 to 6 cups vegetable broth

1½ to 2 cups fresh or frozen cranberries

½ to 1 cup tawny port

INSTRUCTIONS:

Preheat the oven to 350°F.

Place the cubed bread on a baking sheet and bake for about 15 minutes to dry it out. Check frequently to make sure it is not browning too much. Set aside.

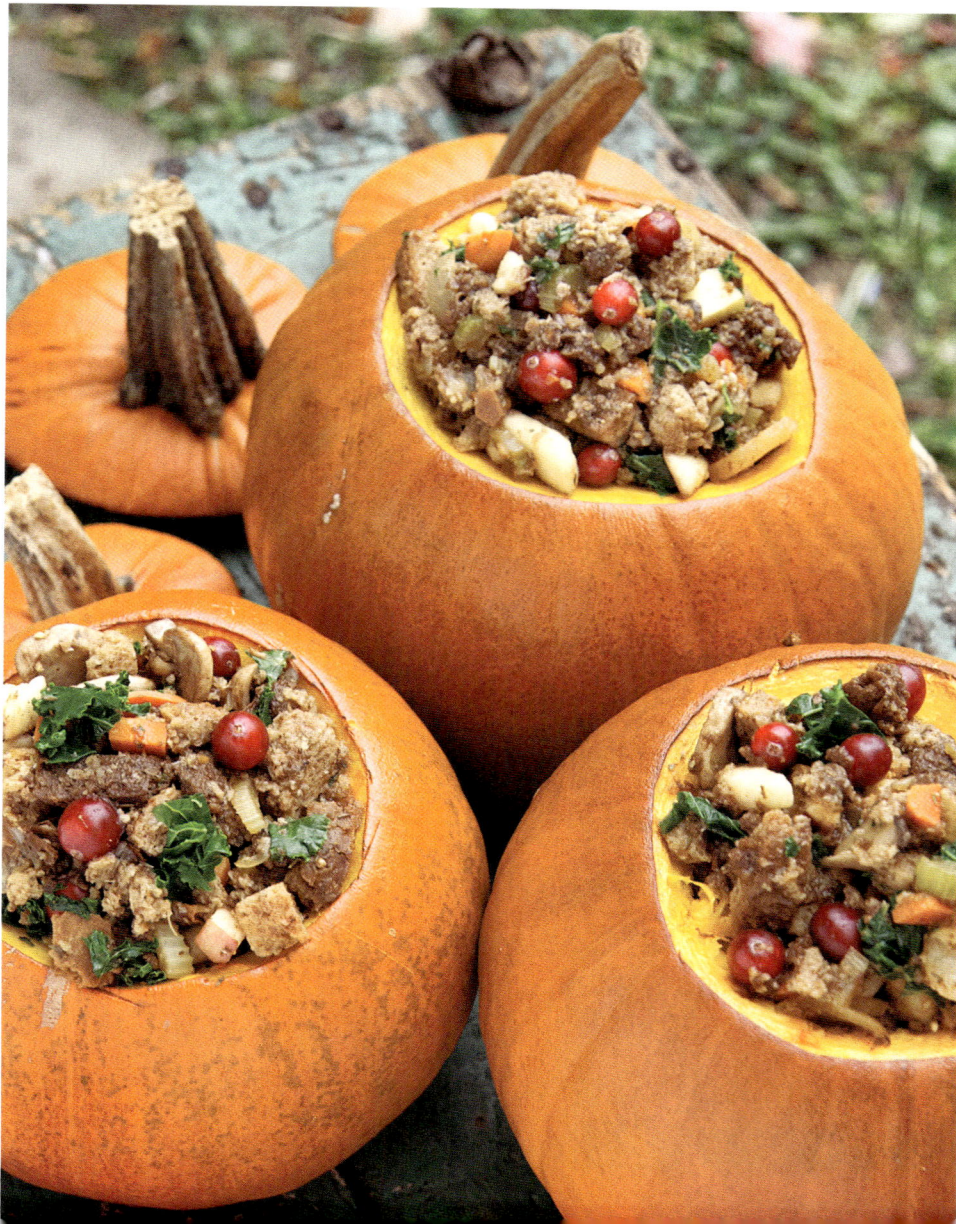

In a frying pan, cook the onion, celery, kale, carrots, and mushrooms over medium-high heat for 8 to 10 minutes until softened. Place the mixture in a large bowl and add the toasted bread cubes, water chestnuts, apples, pear, sage, thyme, oregano, garlic powder, pepper, and cranberries. Add the broth and port to the bowl. Blend and toss until uniformly mixed and soggy. Transfer the moist stuffing to a lasagna pan (or a carved-out pumpkin). Cover with aluminum foil (or the pumpkin lid). Bake for 45 minutes to 1 hour.

Serve warm.

GOOD GARLICKY MASHED POTATOES

You will never believe how good these are until you try them, and you will never believe there is no butter or milk in the recipe. Nothing is as satisfying on a cold day, or if you are just hungry, than a pile of these mashed potatoes! They are delicious plain or with Mommy's Mushroom Gravy 2.0 (page 116), Shiitake Mushroom and Onion Gravy (page 115), or Down Under Cranberry Salsa (page 121). Add greens, if you wish—and by the way, we never peel potatoes.

INGREDIENTS:

6 medium Yukon Gold potatoes

6 tablespoons nutritional yeast

2 teaspoons fresh garlic, minced (2 to 3 cloves)

2 cups nondairy milk of choice (unsweetened almond milk is best here) or water, plus
  more as needed

1 teaspoon dried rosemary

Freshly ground black pepper

½ recipe Cooked Kale (page 23; optional, but a good addition!)

INSTRUCTIONS:

Cut the potatoes into 1-inch chunks and place them into a large pot. Add water to cover and bring the water to a boil. Cook until the potatoes are tender, about 10 minutes. Drain the potatoes, and then place them in a large bowl and mash them.

Add the nutritional yeast, garlic, and nondairy milk, and mash until smooth. They will need more liquid than you might expect since the nutritional yeast soaks up liquid. You may need to add a bit more liquid.

Stir in the rosemary and pepper to taste. Take 1 to 2 cups of the Cooked Kale and chop it into bite-size pieces. Add the kale to the potatoes and gently fold in those little green powerhouses.

JEN'S POTATO SALAD WITH FRESH DILL

SERVES 4 TO 6

A close friend of ours eats no fruit or veggies. None. Shocking, I know. Quite worrisome. So when we arrived for dinner (BYO veggie burgers) and she had this amazing potato salad, I was shocked and thrilled. She said, "Oh, Jane, don't get too excited. Potatoes are tubers and an onion is a bulb. They aren't fruits or vegetables!" The dill in this recipe is my added touch. Jen would not approve of anything green.

INGREDIENTS:

3 pounds red new potatoes, cooked, cooled, and halved or quartered

2 to 3 stalks celery, chopped

6 tablespoons unsweetened applesauce

¼ cup Dijon mustard

½ cup minced shallots

2 tablespoons chopped fresh dill (more or less, to taste)

Freshly ground black pepper

INSTRUCTIONS:

Place the cooked potatoes in a large bowl. In a small bowl, combine the celery, applesauce, Dijon mustard, and shallots, and stir until well combined. Pour the mixture over the potatoes and stir. Add the dill and pepper to taste, toss, and serve.

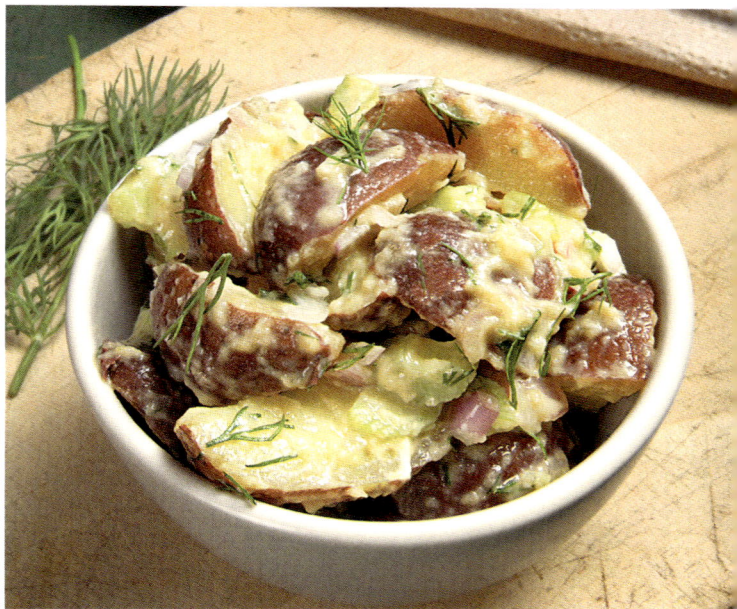

ROASTED RED NEW POTATOES AND GRAVY

Serve this dish warm, alone or with a heaping salad and Cauliflower Steaks (page 233). Be sure to make plenty of Mommy's Mushroom Gravy 2.0 (page 116) or Shiitake Mushroom and Onion Gravy (page 115).

INGREDIENTS:

3 pounds red new potatoes, quartered

2 teaspoons dried rosemary

2 teaspoons dried thyme

1 tablespoon pure maple syrup

½ cup vegetable broth

Mommy's Mushroom Gravy 2.0 (page 115), for serving (optional)

INSTRUCTIONS:

Preheat the oven to 350°F.

Place the potatoes in a roasting pan; add the rosemary, thyme, maple syrup, and broth; and toss until the potatoes are well coated. Roast for 50 minutes until the potatoes are tender. Then turn the oven to broil for the last 10 minutes to brown the potatoes. Serve warm, alone or with Mommy's Mushroom Gravy 2.0.

ZUCCHINI AU GRATIN

The size and number of zucchini in our lives in August overwhelms us. Thus, you may find us feasting on this simple, savory side dish of zucchini and onions for most of that month. We love how tasty and easy it is, not to mention that it puts all of those healthy, hearty, oversize August zucchini to good use.

INGREDIENTS:

- 1 large onion, diced
- 1 large zucchini, cubed (2 to 3 cups)
- 2 to 4 tablespoons nutritional yeast

INSTRUCTIONS:

Heat a large frying pan over high heat until it is so hot that a drop of water forms a bead when dropped in the pan. Add the onion and cook, stirring continuously, while slowly reducing the heat, until the onion is browned and cooked through. Reduce the heat to medium and add the zucchini. Continue to cook, stirring, until the zucchini is cooked to your liking.

Sprinkle with 2 tablespoons of the nutritional yeast to begin with, taste, and add more if you desire. Serve warm.

ZEB'S ROASTED BUTTERNUT SQUASH MEDALLIONS

SERVES 4 TO 6

Our son Zeb has amazed us with this simple, delicious dish. It is impossible to make enough! Look for a butternut squash that is as oblong as possible, which means there may be fewer seeds.

INGREDIENTS:

1 butternut squash

Freshly ground black pepper

Mrs. Dash or other seasoning mix of choice (we recommend Garlic & Herb)

INSTRUCTIONS:

Preheat the oven to 400°F. Line a baking sheet with parchment paper.

With a vegetable peeler, carefully peel the squash, removing all the skin and white so just the bright orange flesh shows.

Slice the squash into ⅛-inch- to ¼-inch-thick medallions (about the thickness of a pencil). On the seeded end, remove the seeds and cut the medallions in half.

Arrange the medallions single file, not overlapping, on the lined pan. Sprinkle with pepper and Mrs. Dash seasoning to taste.

Bake for 20 minutes, until browned but still a little soft inside. Serve as an hors d'oeuvre or colorful vegetable side dish with Eat Loaf (page 184), or with Kale-Lined Tugboats (page 191) and a salad!

TEX-MEX KALE CHIPS

Kale chips are sweeping the world! Our granddaughter's college deli serves them alongside their sandwiches. It's amazing to see. Of course, we are delighted, yet we are also aware of the not-so-healthy ingredients that sometimes make their way into kale chips. So here we have a lean, mean, green Tex-Mex Kale Chip recipe for you!

INGREDIENTS:

8 ounces Our Hummus (page 102) or hummus prepared without oil or tahini

¾ cup nutritional yeast

1 tablespoon Tex-Mex Seasoning made of the following mixed together (save the rest of the Tex-Mex seasoning for other batches of Tex-Mex Kale Chips, or try Penzeys Spices Arizona Dreaming, as it contains no salt):

- ½ tablespoon chili powder
- ½ teaspoon garlic powder
- ½ teaspoon onion powder
- ⅛ teaspoon red pepper flakes
- ¼ teaspoon dried oregano
- ½ teaspoon ground cumin
- ¼ teaspoon freshly ground black pepper, or more to taste

5 to 6 cups kale, stems stripped and leaves torn into bite-size pieces

INSTRUCTIONS:

Preheat the oven to 250°F. (If you want to use dehydrate or convection bake, cooking times will vary, so check your oven manual for comparison to 2 hours baking in a standard oven.) Line two baking sheets with parchment paper.

Combine the hummus, nutritional yeast, Tex-Mex Seasoning, and ⅔ cup water in a medium bowl and mix thoroughly.

Place the kale in a large bowl. Add the sauce to the kale and toss, mixing and tossing the sauce all over and into the contours of the kale leaves.

Spread the well-coated leaves onto the lined baking sheets. Do not stack the leaves on top of one another. Bake the kale chips for 1½ to 2 hours. After 90 minutes, check on the kale chips. Some pieces may be crispy throughout, others may need more time to get crispy, and some may need to be flipped if they are moist underneath. Remove when crisp and dry through and through.

PHILLY-STYLE SOFT PRETZELS

Yes! When we visit Grandpa Eric and Adrienne in Philadelphia, my husband and kids go crazy for the hot, huge, soft Philly pretzels. Here is a healthier version of this favorite treat. Undoubtedly these are best when served hot with mustard! Or dip them into our Sweet-Hot Mustard Dressing and Dip (page 178).

INGREDIENTS:

¾ cup warm water

1 (¼-ounce) packet active dry yeast

2 tablespoons maple syrup

2 cups white whole wheat flour, plus more for kneading

½ cup oat flour

2 tablespoons baking soda

Topping of choice—a sprinkle of whatever you choose: nutritional yeast, poppy seeds, onion flakes, caraway seeds, salt, pepper, or sesame seeds

INSTRUCTIONS:

In a large bowl, mix together the warm water, yeast, maple syrup, and flours. Stir until the dough forms a large clump with an elastic feel.

Divide the dough into 6 equal clumps—each about the size of a small egg—and form them into balls. Place them back in the bowl. Cover the bowl with a damp kitchen towel and let the dough balls rise for at least 25 minutes.

Preheat the oven to 400°F. Line a baking sheet with parchment paper.

Bring a large pot of water to a boil and add the baking soda.

On a lightly floured surface, knead each dough ball, then roll it out into a rope, 12 to 18 inches long. Form a pretzel shape or any other shape you wish. Set the raw pretzel onto a slotted spoon and place it into the boiling water for 10 seconds. Remove the pretzel from the water with the slotted spoon and place it onto the lined baking sheet. While still damp, sprinkle or coat the pretzel with toppings of choice, or nothing at all.

Repeat for the other balls of dough.

When all the pretzels have been boiled and topped (or not!), bake the pretzels for 12 to 15 minutes.

These are best when served hot (they don't have the amazing comfort feel when cold)!

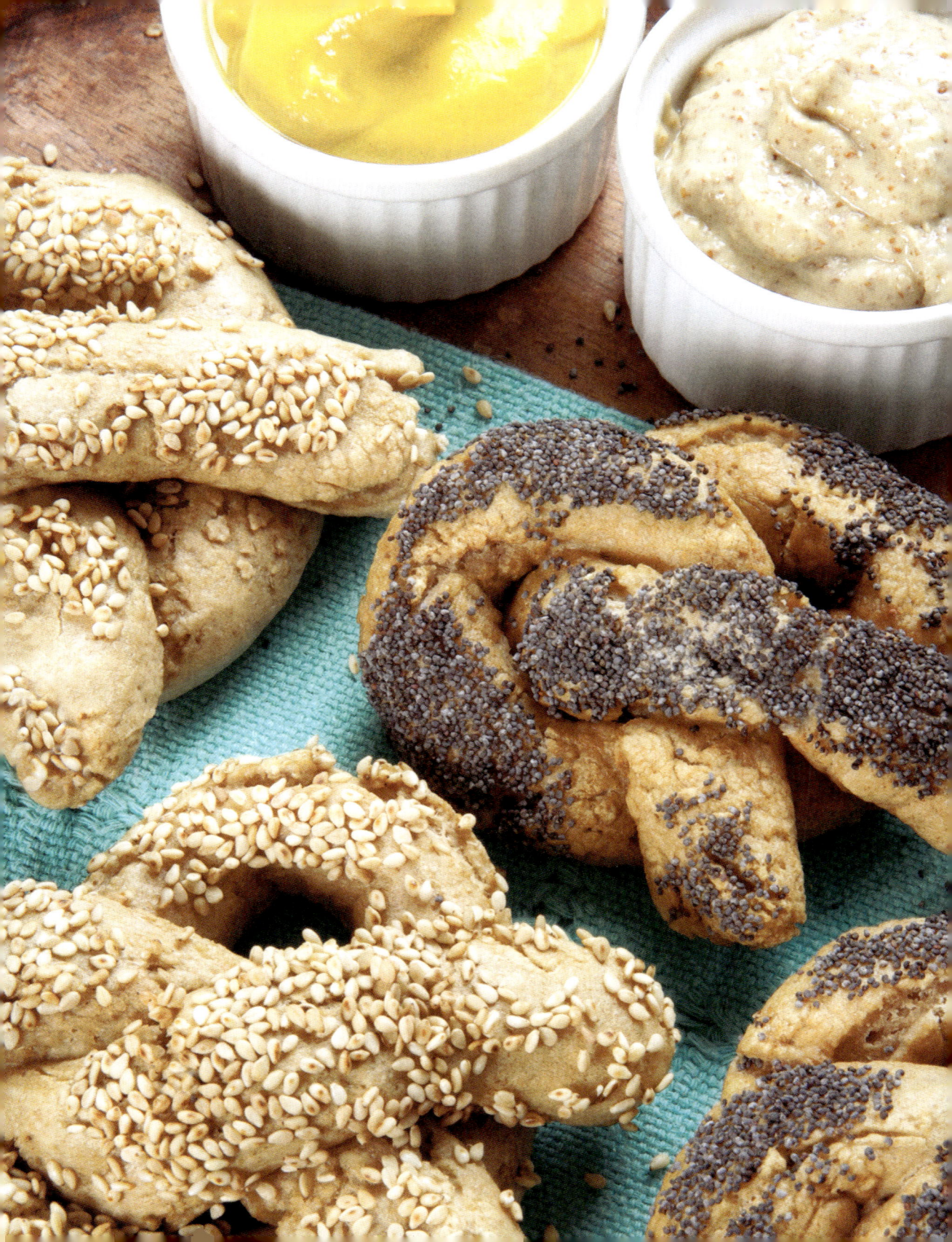

CHEEZY ROUNDS

These have evolved into one of our favorite ways to eat zucchini. We used to have piles of zucchini uneaten from our garden and our CSA (community-supported agriculture) shares. Now we have a war to keep zucchini in the kitchen. And a real battle over these crispy little rounds!

INGREDIENTS:

2 to 3 small zucchini, cut crosswise into rounds ¼ inch thick

½ to ¾ cup nutritional yeast

1 to 2 teaspoons Tex-Mex seasoning, your choice (we recommend Penzeys Spices
    Arizona Dreaming, as it contains no salt) or see Tex-Mex ingredients used in the
    Tex-Mex Kale Chips recipe (page 143)

INSTRUCTIONS:

Preheat the oven to 400°F. Line a baking sheet with parchment paper.

Place the zucchini rounds in a bowl of water.

Mix the nutritional yeast and Tex-Mex seasoning in a small bowl; then put half the mixture in a flat pan or plate with an edge.

Dip both sides of the zucchini in the nutritional yeast mixture and place on the lined baking sheet, using tongs to avoid buildup on your hands from the yeast.

Bake for 30 minutes, or until brown and crisp. Best eaten hot out of the oven!

TATTIES AND NEEPS

Hiking the West Highland Way in Scotland may seem like an impasse for a vegetarian. But I found this dish, and it was a lifesaver! At first I chuckled at the name of the dish, as it sounds like a slang expression my eighth-grade sex ed students might use for certain parts of the female anatomy. But in the Highlands, tatties *are potatoes. And* neeps *are turnips—well, actually, rutabagas (or* swedes*), as they are called in some areas of the UK.*

INGREDIENTS:

3 cups skinned and cubed rutabaga

3 cups cubed potatoes

½ cup plain unsweetened almond or oat milk

¼ cup nutritional yeast

Freshly ground black pepper, to taste

¼ cup fresh parsley, chopped

¼ cup fresh chives chopped (optional)

INSTRUCTIONS:

Place the cubed rutabaga in a large pot of water and bring the water to a boil. After 5 minutes of boiling, add the cubed potatoes to the pot. Cook together for 15 minutes, or until both are quite tender. Drain well.

In the same pot, using a potato masher or a fork, mash the tatties (potatoes) and neeps (turnips/rutabagas/swedes, whatever you want to call them!) together, adding the almond milk, nutritional yeast, and pepper to taste. Stir in the chopped parsley and chives. Serve hot.

ALOO PARATHA–STUFFED INDIAN TORTILLAS

Darshana grew up in a large family in Mumbai absorbing her mother's and aunts' cooking tricks, and now uses her own creativity to make the most wonderful plant-based food. We were lucky to have her in our kitchen for some lessons in Indian cooking. Most of all, we were amazed at how easy and fun it is to make these little stuffed surprises! The recipe below uses traditional Aloo Paratha filling made with potato. Yet we found that mashed cooked sweet potato, or mashed cooked kabocha squash also make good stuffing. Whole wheat flour, which tends to have a higher gluten content than white flour, is necessary for this recipe.

INGREDIENTS:

1½ cups whole wheat flour, plus more for dusting

2 Yukon Gold potatoes or peeled sweet potatoes, cooked and mashed

¼ teaspoon ground turmeric

¼ teaspoon ground cumin

2 tablespoons fresh lime juice

¼ teaspoon garam marsala

2 tablespoons finely chopped green onions

1 tablespoon finely chopped cilantro

Pear-Apple Chutney (page 107) or Mango-Lime Salsa (page 120), for serving

INSTRUCTIONS:

Prepare a large cutting board for rolling out the dough by dusting it with a small amount of whole wheat flour. Place a rolling pin nearby.

Combine the flour and ⅔ cup water in a food processor fitted with a dough blade. Process until it becomes a dough ball, and continue processing the ball for 30 seconds.

Place the mashed potatoes in a bowl add the turmeric, cumin, lime juice, garam masala, green onions, and cilantro, and mash until smooth.

Divide the dough into 6 even portions, 1½ inches in diameter, about the size of a small, flattened potato.

Place one dough ball on the flour-dusted board and roll it on the floured surface, dusting the surface of the ball. With a rolling pin, roll the ball out into a 4-inch-diameter tortilla.

Place about 2 tablespoons of the potato filling in the center of the tortilla and flatten the filling a bit, to 1½ to 2 inches in diameter. Fold the tortilla sides up in a clockwise pattern, one bit at a time to the center where they all meet, so it looks like a beautiful folding coin purse from above.

Using a rolling pin, roll the beautiful filled pocket flat into a 4-inch diameter pancake again.

Place the pancake in a frying pan over medium-low heat and cook until it begins to brown in spots underneath and puff on top. Flip the pancake and cook the other side until it begins to puff as well. Flip the pancake again. Press around the outside edges with a spatula so the outside edges completely cook. Flip it—yes, again—pressing the outside edges with a spatula. Give the pancake one last flip on both sides (each side should cook at least 3 times in the pan).

Repeat with the remaining dough balls and filling. These are best eaten *hot* as they come out of the pan. They are delicious with Pear-Apple Chutney or Mango-Lime Salsa!

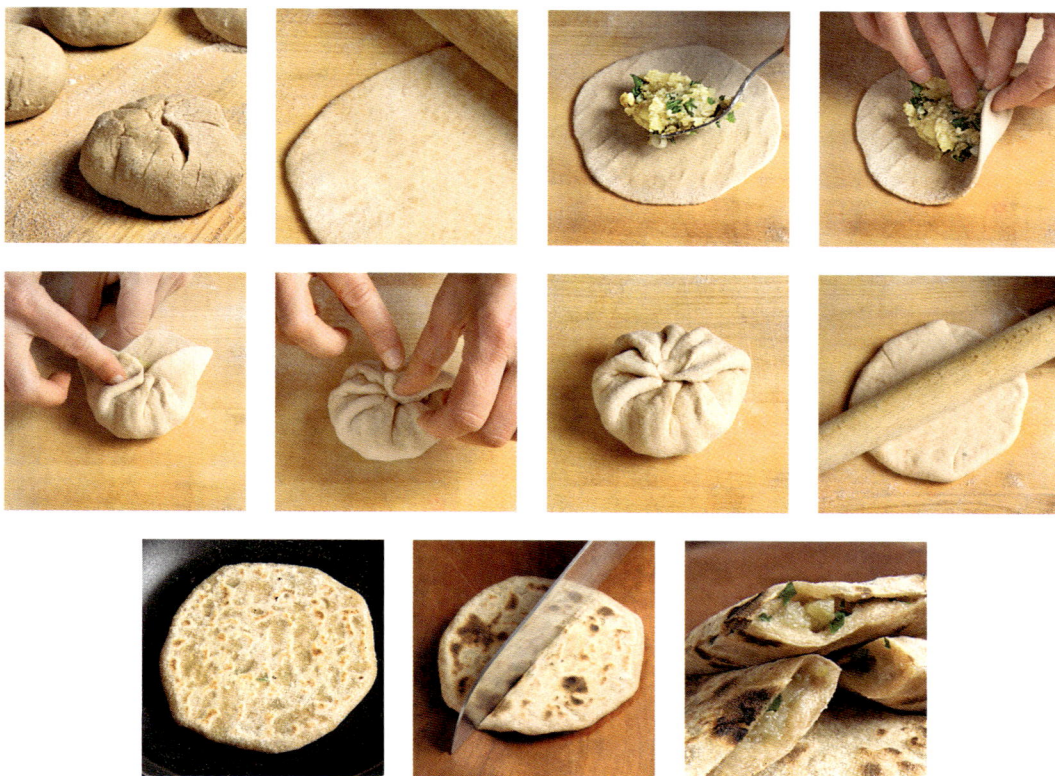

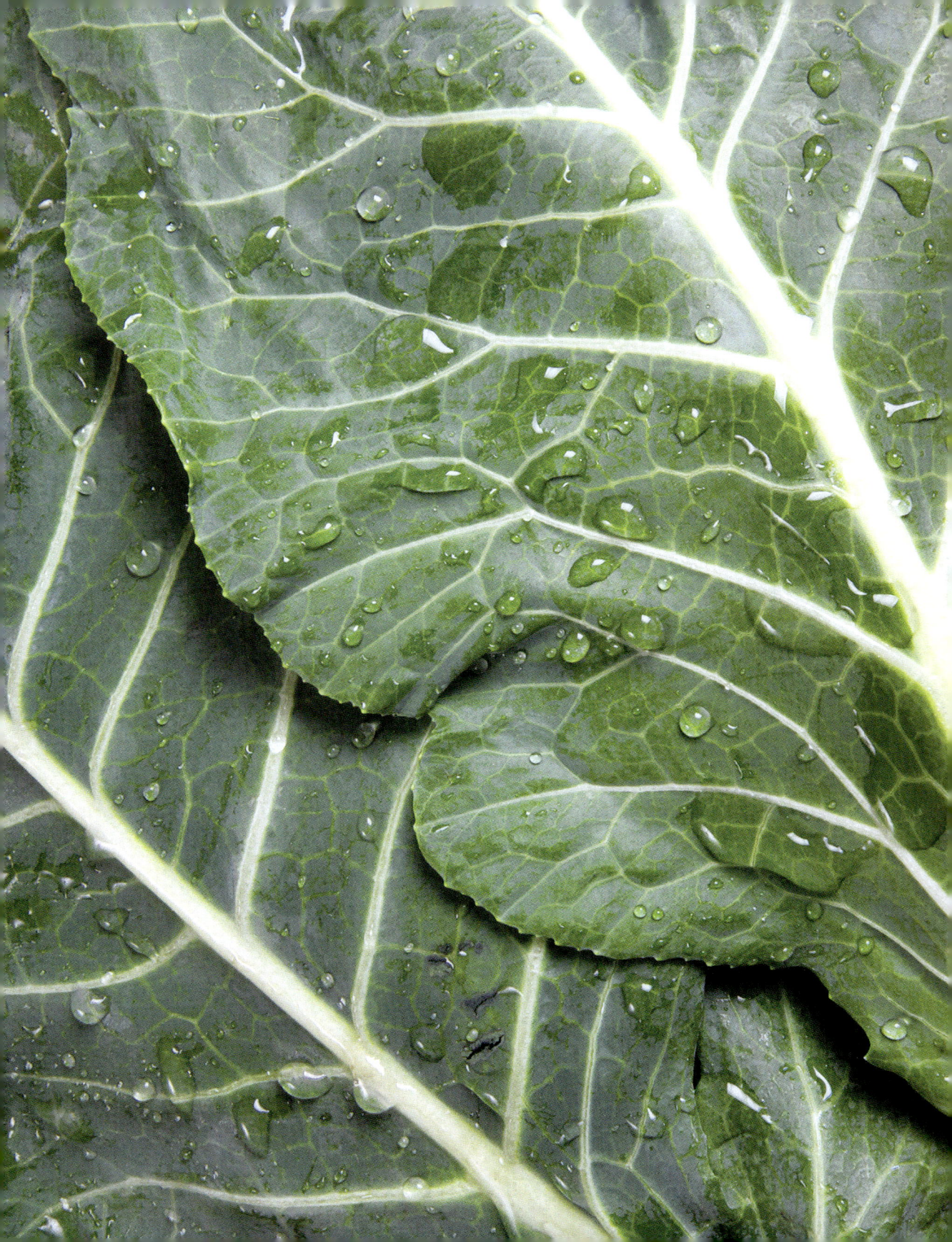

HEARTY SALADS

Oh, salads! Wonderful salads! They can be as simple as a bowl of lettuce or infinitely more complex, and still be the *best* part of a meal. Sometimes they can just be THE MEAL!

Salads are always a part of our dinners. But sometimes we just go for a salad at lunch—with lots of beans and vegetables heaped on top so it's sure to tide us over until dinner. Find a salad dressing you love and it will be easy to relish salads. Dressings can be simple—sometimes just lime juice or a fine balsamic vinegar is all a salad needs. The great thing about salad is you can toss in any vegetables, beans, or fruit you have in your refrigerator—don't be afraid to get creative!

We were at a lunch once and the whole meal was filled with meat, cheese, and creamy sauce, except for one bowl of spinach. I loaded my plate with spinach. The dressing offered was clearly cream-based, but there was a bowl of grapes near the spinach so I piled my spinach with grapes. It was a fabulous new discovery! Every forkful of spinach was so good with a sweet, wet grape. This is all to say, when you are out, there are ways to make surprisingly unorthodox but oddly good choices. When you're eating at home, you can make wildly inventive salads every day of the week.

FRESH FIG AND ARUGULA SALAD

SERVES 2 TO 4

This is so delicious! Fresh figs are in season in early summer and then again in late summer through fall. Choose a slightly soft fig. A good balsamic vinegar, especially one that is fig-infused, is great in this salad and all the dressing it needs (www.olivetap.com is a good website for a wonderful variety of balsamic vinegars, including fig-infused vinegar)! But don't be deterred from making this if you don't have fig balsamic vinegar—any balsamic vinegar works.

INGREDIENTS:

4 fresh figs

6 to 7 cups loosely packed arugula (half of a 5-ounce container)

1 orange

1 tablespoon fig-infused balsamic vinegar or balsamic vinegar of your choice, or to taste

INSTRUCTIONS:

Heat the broiler (it's also easy to do this step in a toaster oven!). Line a small baking pan with aluminum foil. (A toaster oven pan works well.)

Cut the figs in half and place the cut sides down on the lined pan. Broil for 2 minutes. Flip and broil for 2 minutes on the other side.

Place the figs on a cutting board and cut each fig half in half, then in half again.

Place the arugula in a bowl, add the hot figs, and toss.

Cut an orange in half. With a sharp knife, remove the sections and squeeze the juice over the bowl of arugula and figs.

Add the vinegar and mix. Serve while the figs are warm and get ready to receive compliments like, "Oh my, this is so amazing!"

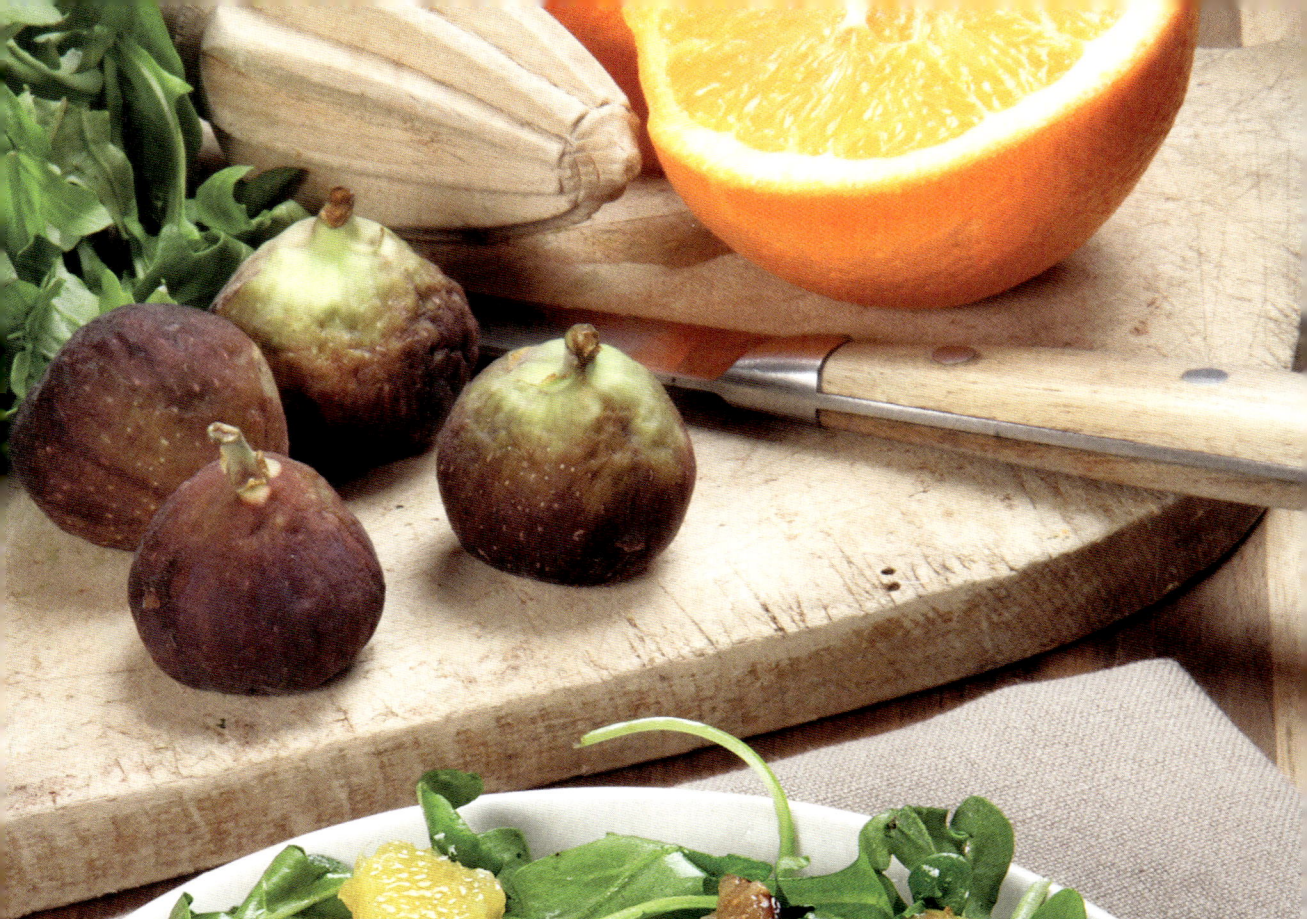

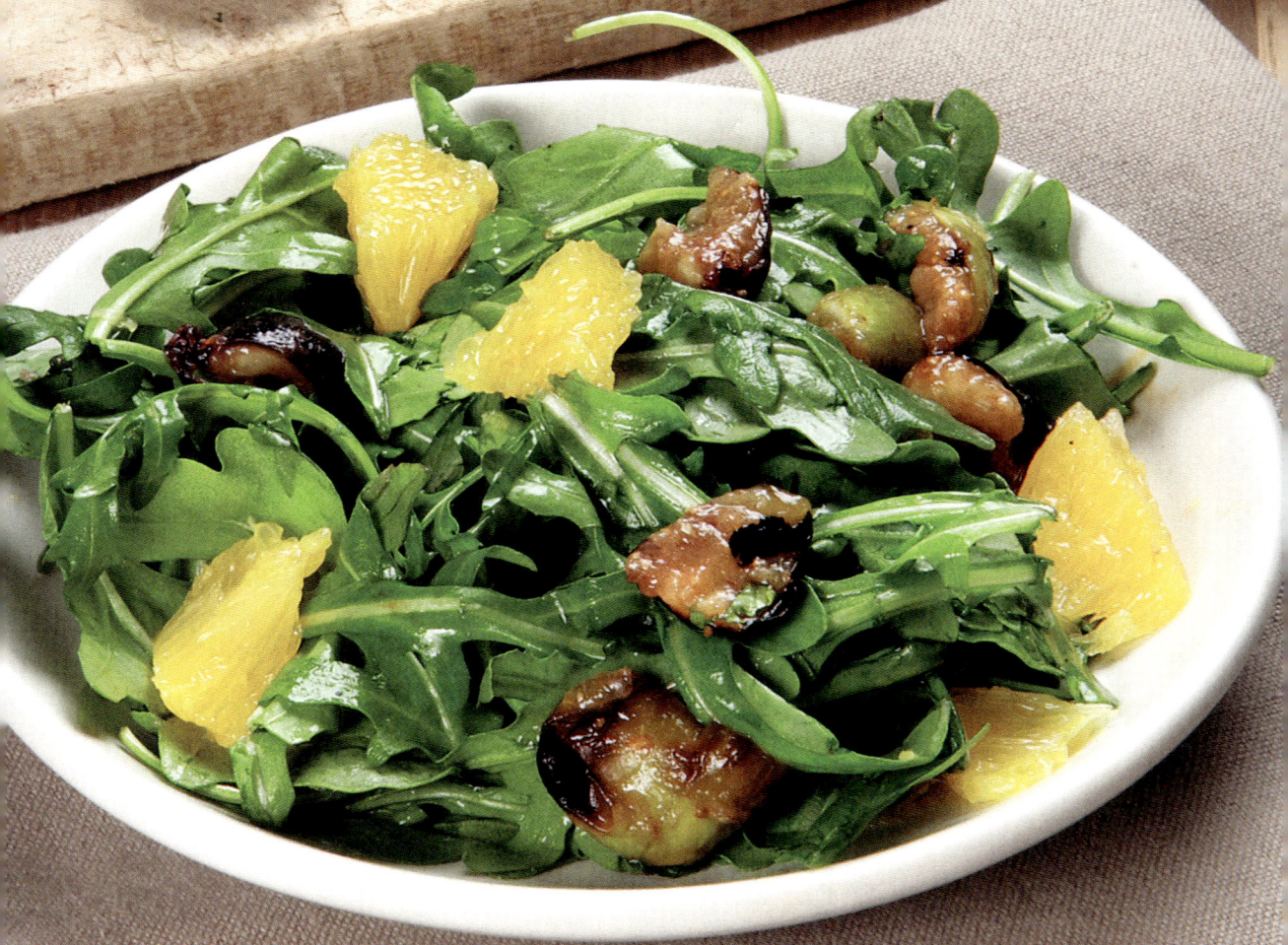

GORGEOUS BLACK RICE SALAD

I made this recipe once when all *our children and grandchildren were arriving from far and wide for dinner. It looked gorgeous and it tasted as good as it looked! Now, it is our new delicious, easy, everyday go-to dish and a real hit for parties! My son-in-law eats this nonstop with Corn Tortilla Taco Shells and Tostados (page 32). It works just as well with brown rice. Try it with white balsamic vinegar if you have some—it tastes the same but looks especially beautiful.*

INGREDIENTS:

2 cups cooked black rice, cooled slightly

1 cup chopped yellow bell pepper

1 cup grape tomatoes, halved

1 cup chopped green onions (about 3), white and green parts

1 cup red grapes, halved

2 cups arugula or spinach

2 mangoes, peeled, pitted, and diced

1 cup chopped fresh cilantro

2 tablespoons balsamic vinegar, or to taste

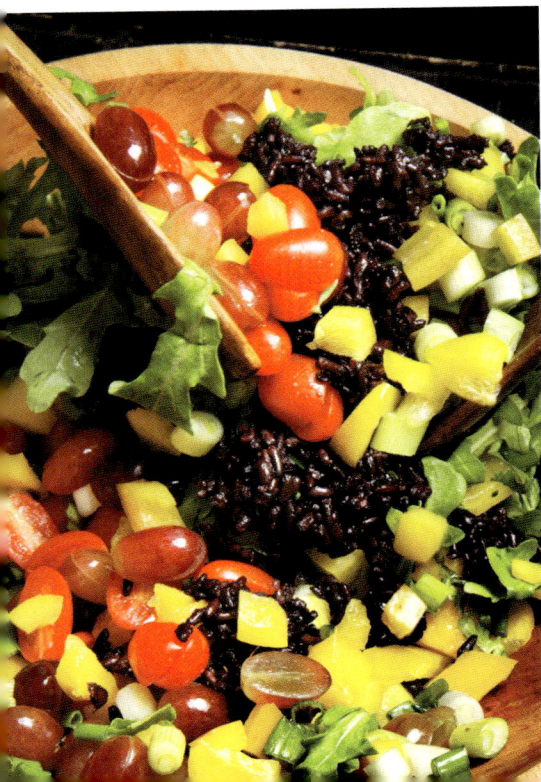

INSTRUCTIONS:

Place the cooked rice in a large, broad bowl. Add the bell pepper, tomatoes, green onions, grapes, arugula, 1½ of the mangoes, and the cilantro, and toss gently.

In a food processor or high-speed blender, combine the remaining mango half and the balsamic vinegar. Blend until smooth and pour over the rice and vegetables. Toss to coat before serving.

FRENCH LENTILS WITH GRAPES AND MINT

SERVES 3 TO 4

Oh, this is a good combination of tastes! Olive Tap (www.olivetap.com) makes fabulous balsamic vinegars in many, many flavors . . . black currant, tangerine, Sicilian lemon, etc. One of our favorites is their traditional balsamic vinegar. We use it on this salad—a delicious balsamic is all it needs for perfection. Add more vinegar if you find the lentils too dry.

INGREDIENTS:

2 cups cooked French lentils

2 cups red grapes, halved

¼ cup mint, chopped

⅓ cup parsley, chopped

2 tablespoons good balsamic vinegar

Arugula, spinach, or other greens, for serving

INSTRUCTIONS:

Combine the cooked lentils, grapes, mint, parsley, and balsamic vinegar in a bowl. Stir gently and serve on a bed of arugula, spinach, or other greens of your choice.

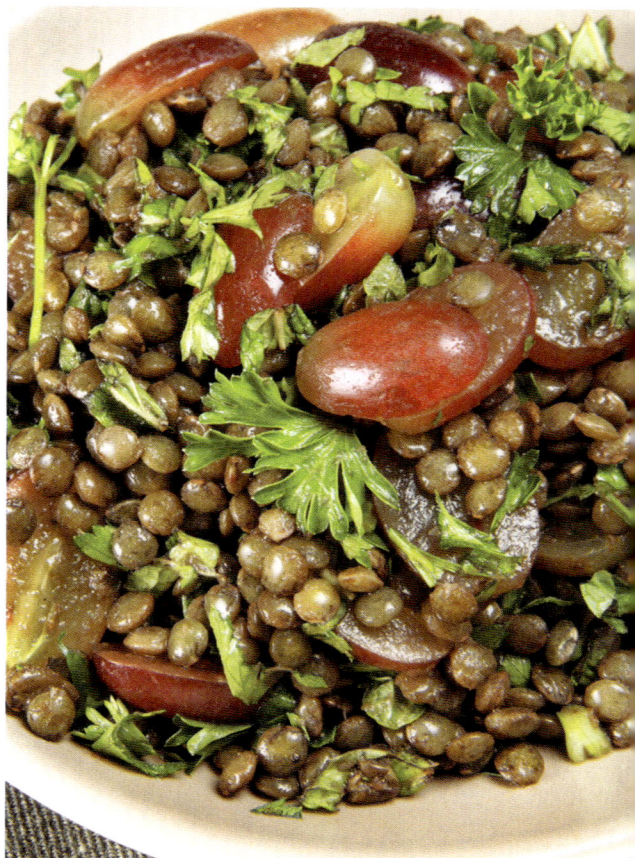

BEETS AND BEET GREENS WITH DIJON DRIZZLE

Beets and mustard! Our daughter-in-law Polly told us about this delicious combination. To make this salad a hearty, whole meal, serve the beets and greens on top of farro or rice. If you don't have enough beet greens, Swiss chard works well and looks very similar. If you are in a hurry, forget the mushrooms, boil the greens for a few minutes until they are soft, drain, and continue as below. For a spectacular presentation, serve this in Crispy Tortilla Bowls (page 30). You will wow everyone!

INGREDIENTS:

1 bunch beets with greens attached (about 4 beets and 2 cups greens)

2 cloves garlic, chopped

3½ ounces fresh shiitake mushrooms

2 tablespoons Dijon mustard

1 teaspoon pure maple syrup

INSTRUCTIONS:

To prepare the beets, cut the greens off where the stems meet the bulb, reserving the greens. Trim the ends of the beets and discard.

Cook the beets either way you prefer: Boil them in enough water to cover for about 50 minutes, until fork-tender, or wrap them in aluminum foil and bake at 425°F for an hour, or until they are easily pricked with a fork.

Allow the beets to cool; then peel off the skin of the beets. (We love this peeling part.)

Slice the beets into rounds. If your beets are large, cut the rounds in half, and set aside.

In a frying pan, cook the garlic over medium heat in a little water until translucent. Add the shiitake mushrooms and cook until wilted. Add more water as needed in small drops as it evaporates.

Clean the beet greens well and chop the leaves and stems into bite-size pieces. Add the greens and stems to the pan with the garlic and mushrooms and continue to cook until the greens wilt and the stems soften.

In a small saucepan, combine the Dijon mustard, maple syrup, and 2 tablespoons water, and cook over low heat until warm. (This dressing does not need to be served warm.)

On each individual plate, arrange a portion of cooked beet greens and stems. Then add a layer of sliced beet rounds. Drizzle all over with the mustard dressing.

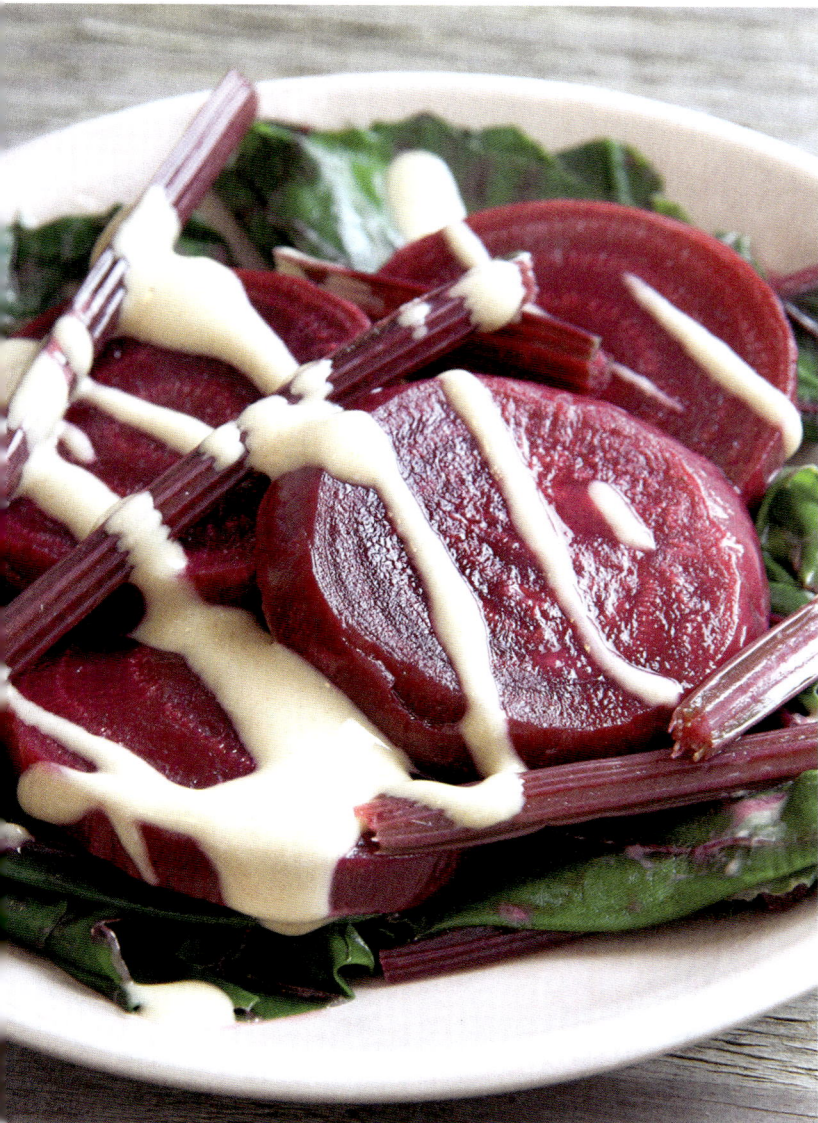

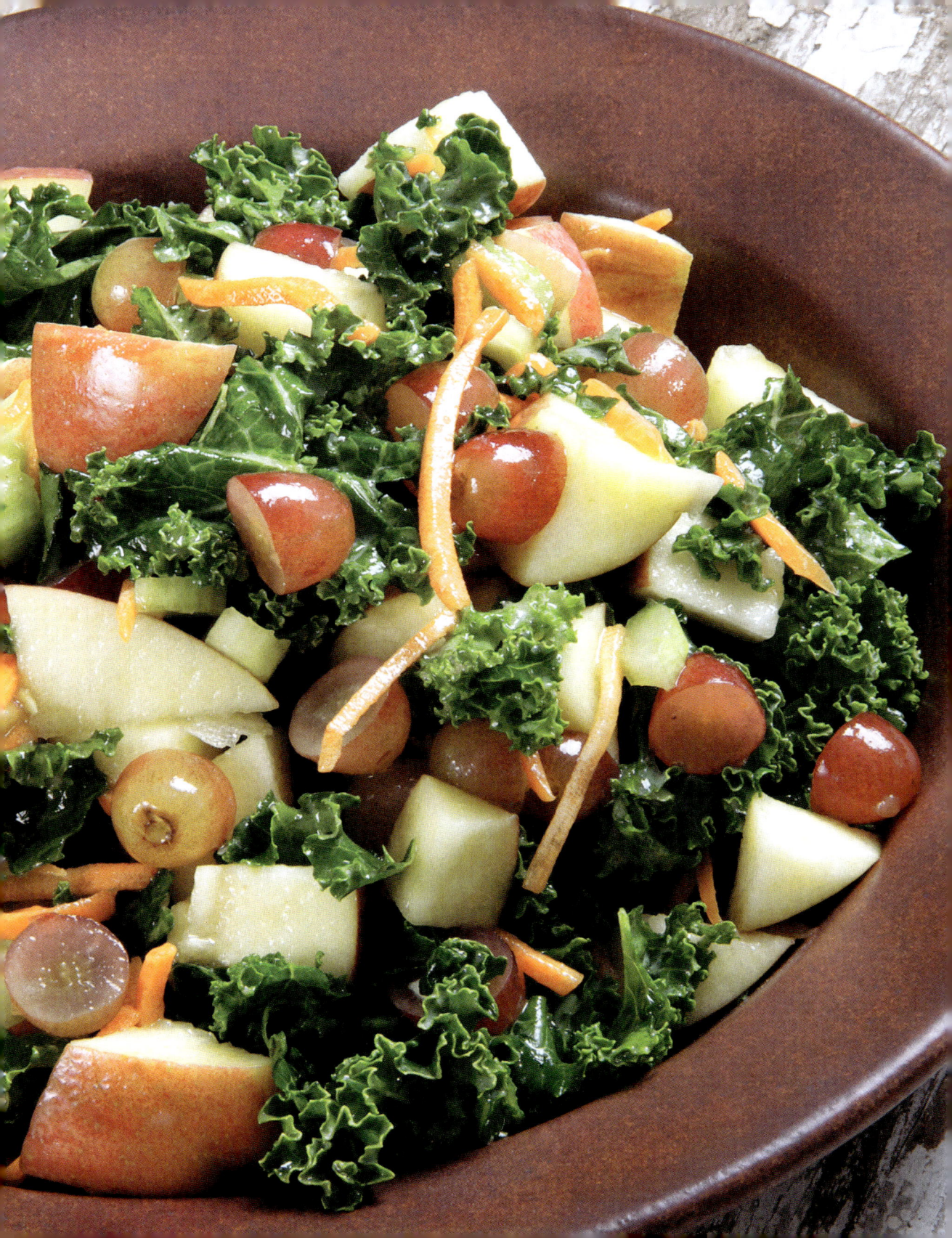

KALE WALDORF SALAD

This recipe seems to be the talk of the plant-based town. The same week a friend told us she'd had this salad in Santa Fe, New Mexico, we got this recipe from an amazing plant-based restaurant in Tucson, Arizona, called Lovin' Spoonfuls. The banana and vinegar combine here in a surprisingly delicious way. We have added some kale, of course. We like to serve it over a bed of butter lettuce, or, for a heartier meal, try it over brown basmati rice.

INGREDIENTS:

- ½ ripe banana
- 2 teaspoons apple cider vinegar
- 2 cups kale, stems removed and leaves torn into bite-size pieces
- 2 apples, cored and diced
- 1 stalk celery, diced
- ½ cup red grapes, halved
- ½ cup shredded carrots
- Ground cinnamon, for sprinkling

INSTRUCTIONS:

In a food processor, combine the banana and the vinegar and process until smooth.

Place the kale in a large bowl and pour the banana mixture over the kale. Massage the dressing into the kale with your hands until the kale turns dark green and relaxes a bit.

Add the apples, celery, grapes, and carrots, and toss.

Sprinkle with cinnamon, cover, and chill for at least 30 minutes. Serve chilled.

REBOOT SALAD

This salad is inspired by a Whole Foods Market's "detox" salad. I just love it—not for its detox power but for the burst of energy it gives. Thus, we are calling this Reboot Salad! It is loaded with vitamins C and K, beta-carotene, iron, calcium, and fiber. What a reboot! Make sure to chop the vegetables into tiny, tiny pieces. That is the key to what makes this salad so tasty. It tastes amazing with raisin-lemon dressing and can be scooped up with crispy Tostados (page 32).

INGREDIENTS:

3 cups broccoli, chopped into tiny pea-size pieces

3 cups cauliflower, chopped into tiny pea-size pieces

1 cup carrots, shredded and chopped into tiny pieces

3 stalks celery, minced fine

1½ cups parsley, minced fine

1½ cups raisins

¾ cup fresh lemon juice

Freshly ground black pepper

2 tablespoons sesame seeds, toasted

INSTRUCTIONS:

In a salad bowl, combine the broccoli, cauliflower, carrots, celery, and parsley.

Place the raisins in a small bowl and add 1½ cups hot water. After 5 minutes of soaking, drain the water off the raisins and reserve it.

In a food processor, combine the raisins, lemon juice, and 1 cup of the reserved raisin soaking water, and blend until smooth. Add pepper to taste.

Pour the raisin-lemon dressing over the vegetables and toss well. Sprinkle the sesame seeds on top, serve it up, and step high!

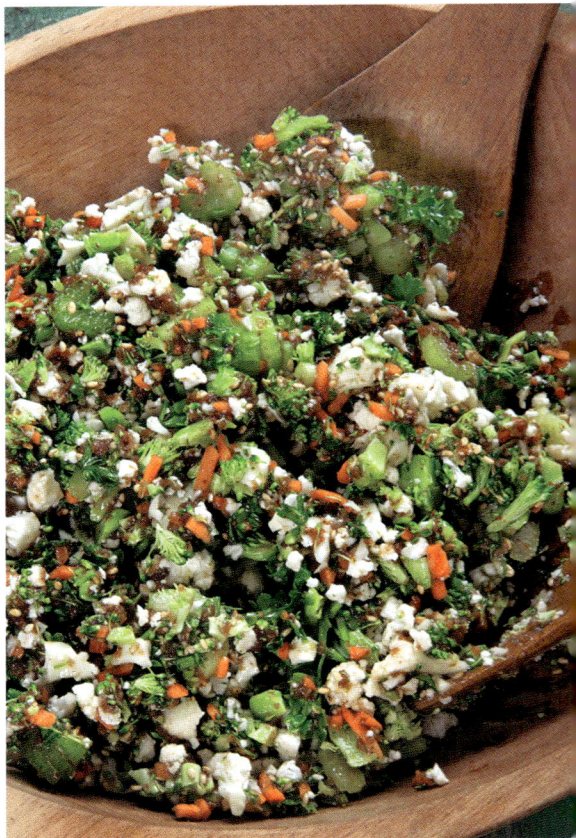

BLACK BEAN SUCCOTASH SALAD

Black bean salads are a favorite in our family. We could eat them at every meal of the day, especially in the summer! This recipe combines things we love—lima beans, black beans, artichokes, water chestnuts—that crazily work well together. Artichokes are a family special-occasion food. And, of course, we can't live without balsamic vinegar! It is easy to expand this salad by adding more beans, corn, or tomatoes. Or be adventurous and add anything from your garden. If you are using frozen vegetables, it is an easy trick to thaw them under warm running water.

INGREDIENTS:

2 (15-ounce) cans no-salt-added black beans, drained and rinsed

2 tomatoes, cored and chopped

16 ounces frozen corn, thawed, or kernels from about 5 ears of fresh corn

16 ounces frozen baby lima beans, thawed

1 can artichoke bottoms, diced

1 (8-ounce) can sliced water chestnuts

4 green onions, chopped

½ onion, chopped

3 tablespoons lemon juice

Zest of 1 lemon

3 tablespoons balsamic vinegar

INSTRUCTIONS:

Combine the black beans, tomatoes, corn, lima beans, artichokes, water chestnuts, green onions, and onions in a large bowl and stir.

Add the lemon juice, lemon zest, and balsamic vinegar to the salad and stir again. Serve!

QUINOA TABBOULEH

In the 1970s, tabbouleh was the weird food our yogi-loving neighbor ate all the time. Now it is a dish we eat all the time, and we love yoga now, too. Try it stuffed into a whole wheat pita or Corn Tortilla Taco Shells and Tostados (page 32) with some spinach, and have it to go!

INGREDIENTS:

1½ cups cooked quinoa

2 cups cherry tomatoes, quartered

1 medium cucumber, diced (about 2 cups)

1 (15-ounce) can no-salt-added chickpeas, drained and rinsed

2 cloves garlic, minced

½ small red onion, diced

4 cups very, very finely chopped parsley

¼ cup mint leaves, minced

6 tablespoons fresh lemon juice

½ teaspoon freshly ground black pepper

3 tablespoons white balsamic vinegar

¼ teaspoon ground cumin

Butter lettuce or other greens of your choice, for serving

INSTRUCTIONS:

In a large bowl, combine the quinoa, tomatoes, cucumber, chickpeas, garlic, onion, parsley, mint, lemon juice, pepper, balsamic vinegar, and cumin, and stir. Refrigerate until ready to serve. The flavors bloom together the longer you wait. Serve over butter lettuce or other greens of your choice.

LIGHT ASIAN SLAW

This is light and bright and out of sight! It is summer on a fork and won't weigh you down a bit. We love it with Pacific Rim Soba Noodles (page 190). Make sure the cubes of mango are very small—about the size of the tip of your pinkie finger.

INGREDIENTS:

3 cups Napa cabbage, finely shredded

2 cups cubed mango (the juicier, the better)

2 teaspoons grated, peeled fresh ginger

Zest and juice of 1 lime

INSTRUCTIONS:

Combine the cabbage and mango in a salad bowl.

In a small bowl, combine the ginger, lime zest, and lime juice.

Add the ginger dressing to the cabbage and mango. Toss with your hands to spread the dressing uniformly.

Serve immediately or chill until ready to eat.

MASSAGED KALE SALAD WITH MANGO AND LIME

SERVES 4 TO 6

Everyone has been raving about kale salad massaged with avocado. Our daughter-in-law Anne had the idea to use hummus instead of avocado! Oh my goodness, it was a hit the first time around! It is amazing what a little massaging does for kale; it becomes tender, dark, and easier to chew. You can make a quick version of this salad if you just massage the kale with hummus and lemon and simply add lemon juice and cherry tomatoes. Mango, mint, and lime take it to a totally new level of deliciousness.

INGREDIENTS:

1 bunch kale, stems stripped and leaves torn into bite-size pieces

¼ cup Our Hummus (page 102) or hummus prepared without oil or tahini

Zest of ½ to 1 lime

2 tablespoons fresh lime juice, or more to taste

1 mango, pitted, peeled, and cubed

2 cups frozen corn, thawed

1 to 2 cups cherry tomatoes, halved (choose yellow, if available)

1 yellow bell pepper, seeded and chopped

2 tablespoons fresh mint, chopped

INSTRUCTIONS:

Place the kale in a large salad bowl and with your hands massage the hummus into the kale. It will soften quickly. Keep massaging until the kale is limp and well coated. The more you massage, the more tender, dark, and edible the kale becomes!

Add the lime zest and lime juice, and stir. Add more hummus or lime juice to taste.

Add the mango, corn, tomatoes, yellow bell pepper, and mint, and toss gently. Yum—this is a winner!

TED'S HOUSE SALAD

Everyone wants to be like Ted: He is an artist, a carpenter, savior of urban hardwoods, a designer of kids' museums, and an MD. Somehow between carpooling his three kids around town, he does as much in one day as three men his size. His world, his home, and his work are beautiful, colorful, and chaotic—just tons of fun. His fridge is the same. Making a salad at his house feels like nutritional art class. He always has different types of greens, berries, jicama, purple peppers, and a bazillion different huge, colored salad bowls with wacky tongs. Here is a typical salad from Ted's house.

INGREDIENTS:

- 3 cups spring greens
- ½ jicama, peeled and cut into strips
- 2 carrots, sliced
- 1 purple bell pepper or red bell pepper, seeded and cut into strips
- ½ English cucumber, sliced
- 2 purple potatoes or red new potatoes, cooked and sliced
- ¼ cup raspberries
- 1 small apple, cut into thin horizontal circles with the beautiful center star featured
- ½ cup raisins
- ¼ cup pumpkin seeds, toasted (optional)

TED'S HOUSE DRESSING INGREDIENTS:

- 2 to 3 tablespoons hummus prepared without oil or tahini
- 2 tablespoons vinegar (more or less to taste)
- 1 tablespoon pure maple syrup (to taste)
- Splash of orange juice

INSTRUCTIONS:

Combine the greens, jicama, carrots, peppers, cucumber, potatoes, raspberries, apple, raisins, and pumpkin seeds (if using) in a funky bowl, dress, and serve with wacky tongs.

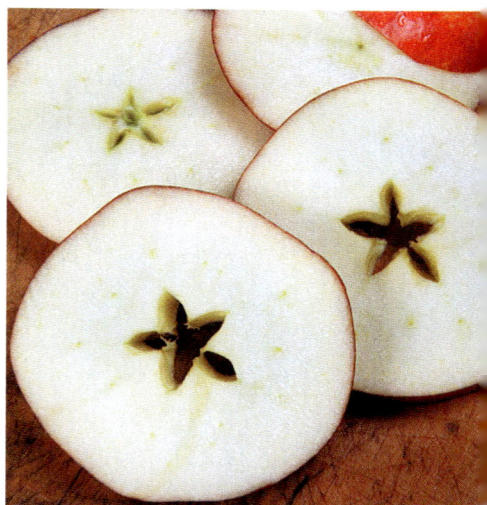

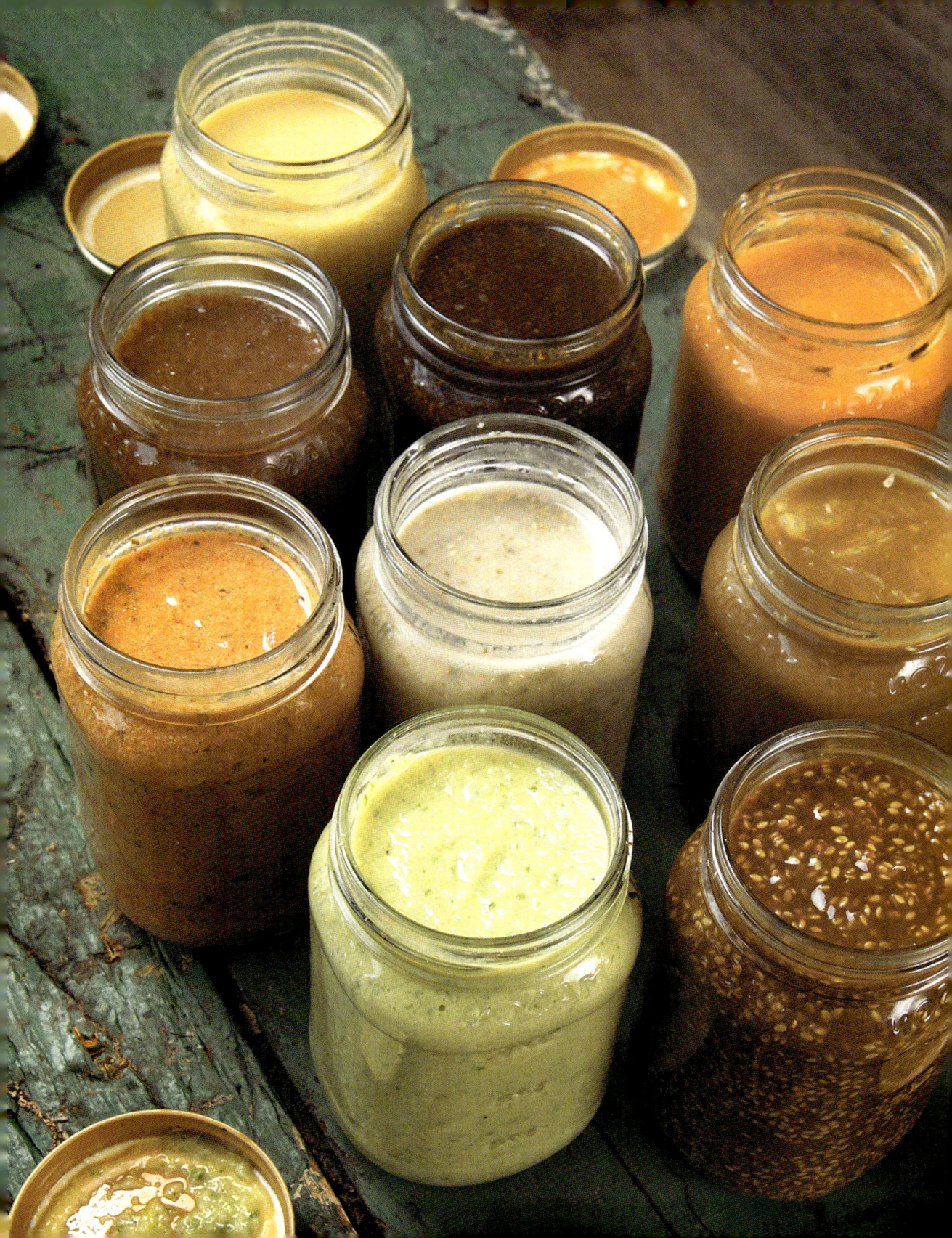

SALAD DRESSINGS

There is *nothing* harder than finding a salad dressing you love! It took us a long time, but we found one we love that we use on everything nearly every day. Experiment and experiment until you find one you love, too. Be confident. It will happen, and you will *never* look back on those old days when you used oil.

The salad dressing game-changer for us happened a number of years ago when a friend gave us the present of Black Currant Balsamic Vinegar from the Olive Tap (www.olivetap.com). Since then, we have become Olive Tap first-name-basis customers. We love their amazing varieties of vinegars. Though it's a hard call, our favorites are Black Currant and their original 4 Leaf. Many people find these vinegars alone are the solution to salad dressings. We hear raves about White Orange from a number of patients, but equal enthusiasm about Tangerine, Fig, Lemon, Peach, Raspberry, etc. There are a number of different Olive Tap stores across the country. If there is a store near you, take advantage and go taste the amazing variety they offer. But many specialty supermarkets offer high-end and delicious balsamic vinegar brands, and some offer tastings of them as well. Conveniently, many balsamic vinegar companies carry small jars, which are easy to carry in your purse or a bag when you need a quick, good dressing while you are out!

ANN AND ESSY'S FAVORITE DRESSING

This is the secret recipe in the book. Really, it is. My parents have this every day. This is what courses through their veins. We share this recipe with high hopes that you will find your own favorite dressing—as that truly is the key to happily devouring salads. Find a recipe you love, make loads of it. Keep it in your fridge door at home, at work, and even at your in-laws'!

INGREDIENTS:

2 tablespoons Our Hummus (page 102) or hummus prepared without oil or tahini

2 tablespoons fresh orange juice, or sections from ½ orange and their juice

2 tablespoons balsamic vinegar

2 teaspoons mustard, your favorite

1 teaspoon minced peeled fresh ginger

INSTRUCTIONS:

In a small bowl, combine the hummus, orange juice, balsamic vinegar, mustard, and ginger with a fork. Toss onto your salad and enjoy.

VARIATION:

Add 1 tablespoon nutritional yeast to the mix!

BIRTHDAY DRESSING

My husband and father have birthdays very close together; thus, we have a combined party and feast. I made this dressing for the party this year, and my father liked it so much he poured it over everything on his plate!

INGREDIENTS:

- 3 tablespoons balsamic glaze (we prefer Isola Classic Cream of Balsamic)
- 2 tablespoons mustard, your choice
- Juice of ½ lime
- ¼ cup sesame seeds, toasted (be careful not to burn them; I always do!)

INSTRUCTIONS:

In a bowl, combine the balsamic glaze, mustard, and lime juice, and stir.
Add the sesame seeds, stir again, and serve.

GINGER-LEMON SALAD DRESSING

This is fabulous, smooth, delicious, and lemony. If you want a lighter-colored salad dressing, use white balsamic vinegar. For a wonderful added lemon flavor, use lemon balsamic vinegar (it's white), available at www.olivetap.com. Any white beans will work, but cannellini are the smoothest. Try this on Ted's House Salad (page 165) or on any green salad.

INGREDIENTS:

1 (15-ounce) can no-salt-added cannellini beans, drained and rinsed

1 tablespoon capers, rinsed and drained

1 large clove garlic, chopped

2 tablespoons lemon juice plus zest of 1 lemon

1 tablespoon minced peeled fresh ginger

¼ cup balsamic vinegar

Freshly ground black pepper

INSTRUCTIONS:

Put the beans, capers, garlic, lemon juice, lemon zest, and ginger in a food processor, and process until smooth. Add the balsamic vinegar and 6 tablespoons water, and continue to blend until uniformly smooth. Season to taste with pepper.

RAISIN-LEMON DRESSING

This is a sweet surprise of a dressing. We love it on the Reboot Salad (page 160). Give your iron levels a boost with this yummy raisin-based dressing.

INGREDIENTS:

1½ cups raisins

¾ cup fresh lemon juice

Freshly ground black pepper

INSTRUCTIONS:

Place the raisins in a small bowl and add 1½ cups hot water. Set aside to soak for 5 minutes. Drain the raisins, reserving the soaking water.

Place the raisins in a high-speed blender or food processor with the lemon juice and 1 cup of the reserved raisin soaking water, and blend until smooth. Add pepper to taste.

HOT STUFF DRESSING

This dressing makes a salad feel like more of a meal. It is savory and flavor-y and packs some heat. Bang! Bang! Try this over Cooked Kale (page 23) or on any spinach salad you create.

INGREDIENTS:

- ½ cup nutritional yeast
- ½ cup prepared salsa
- ½ teaspoon chili powder
- ¼ teaspoon red pepper flakes
- ¼ teaspoon garlic powder
- ½ teaspoon onion powder
- ¼ cup water
- Pinch of cayenne

INSTRUCTIONS:

In a bowl, combine the nutritional yeast, salsa, chili powder, red pepper flakes, garlic powder, onion powder, water, and cayenne, and mix well. You can vary the amounts of the cayenne and nutritional yeast according to your taste.

SUSIE CUKE DRESSING

My sister Susan Crile is not only an outstanding artist but also a creative cook. This cucumber dressing of hers is one of our favorites—she's really perfected it. It is light and goes beautifully on Bibb lettuce, romaine, arugula, spring greens—or really anything!

INGREDIENTS:

½ English cucumber, chopped

2 cloves garlic

⅛ teaspoon freshly ground black pepper

1 tablespoon Dijon mustard

2 tablespoons fresh lemon juice

¾ cup Our Hummus (page 102) or hummus prepared without oil or tahini

¼ cup brown rice vinegar

1 tablespoon white balsamic vinegar

INSTRUCTIONS:

In a food processor, combine the cucumber, garlic, pepper, Dijon mustard, lemon juice, hummus, rice vinegar, and balsamic vinegar, and process until smooth. Serve fresh or, if necessary, refrigerate in an airtight container until ready to use.

JANE'S FAVORITE 3, 2, 1 DRESSING

MAKES ⅓ CUP

The 3, 2, 1 base of this dressing is the key. Then, sometimes I add different flavors to spice it up! This recipe is in My Beef with Meat *and* Prevent and Reverse Heart Disease. *It is such a winner. Below is my favorite version by far.*

INGREDIENTS:

- 3 tablespoons balsamic vinegar
- 2 tablespoons mustard of choice
- 1 tablespoon pure maple syrup
- Juice of 1 lemon
- Pinch of freshly ground white pepper (optional)

INSTRUCTIONS:

Combine all the ingredients in a small bowl with a whisk until smooth. Serve over salad or greens.

CITRUS SALAD DRESSING

This is a nice summer dressing—so light, so fresh. Use this on all of summer's beautiful lettuces. It's especially good with a green salad filled with fresh raspberries and orange slices.

INGREDIENTS:

3 tablespoons fresh orange juice

Zest and juice of 1 lime

1 to 2 teaspoons pure maple syrup

6 mint leaves, cut into chiffonade

INSTRUCTIONS:

Combine the orange juice, lime zest, lime juice, syrup, and mint, and stir with a whisk to combine.

MANGO SALAD DRESSING

MAKES ABOUT 1 CUP

This is absolutely delicious, so easy, and adds a wonderful just-right sweetness to a salad. To keep the dressing a beautiful orange, use white balsamic vinegar, if possible.

INGREDIENTS:

1 mango, pitted, peeled, and roughly chopped

¼ cup balsamic vinegar, preferably white

INSTRUCTIONS:

Place the mango chunks and vinegar in a food processor and process until smooth.

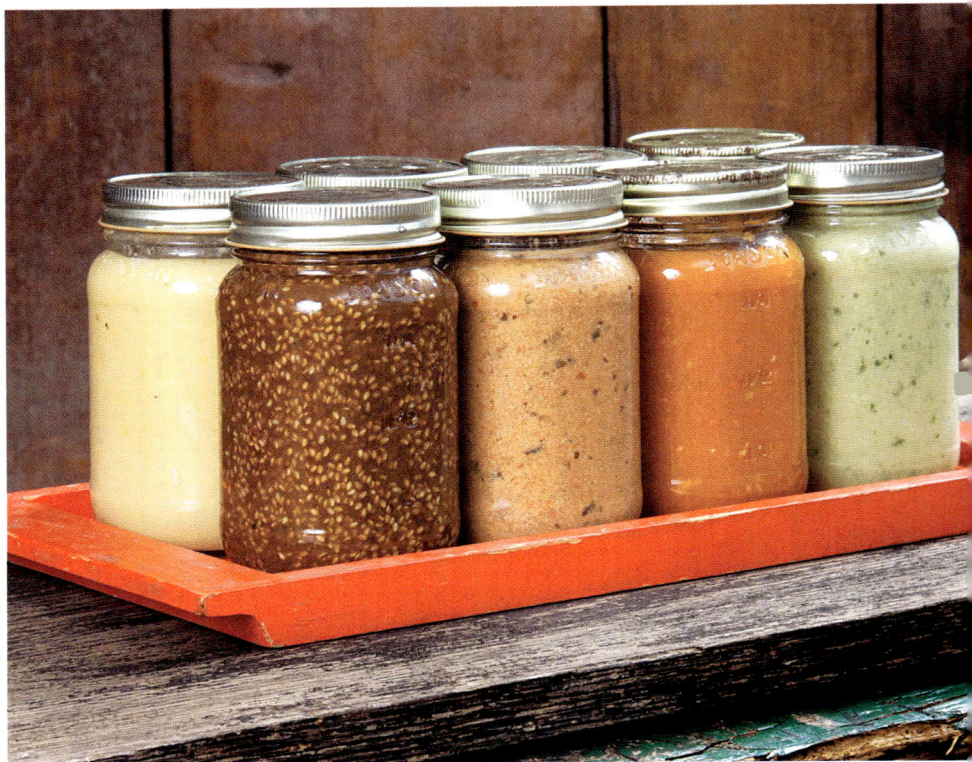

LEMONETTE

This dressing totally satisfies my lemon love and is delicious on anything. We especially like it on kale that has been well massaged with hummus. The idea for this dressing is from chef JP Iacobucci, executive chef at Martini Modern Italian in Columbus, Ohio. A good white balsamic vinegar is important. We like Acetaia Cattani or Olive Tap's white balsamic vinegars.

INGREDIENTS:

Zest of ½ lemon

2 tablespoons fresh lemon juice

2 tablespoons white balsamic vinegar

Freshly ground black pepper

INSTRUCTIONS:

In a small bowl, combine the lemon zest, lemon juice, balsamic vinegar, and pepper to taste. Stir and get ready for that amazing zing!

SWEET-HOT MUSTARD DRESSING AND DIP

Sometimes friends bring over the best dishes. It leaves you wondering why you bothered to cook when everything the guest brings is so fantastic. A friend brought this dressing over once and I haven't stopped loving it on everything: salads, grains, greens, and my Philly-Style Soft Pretzels (page 144). Beware: This is a hottie!

INGREDIENTS:

- ½ cup plain oat milk
- ½ to 1 teaspoon cayenne pepper
- ¼ cup Dijon mustard or spicy brown mustard
- ¼ cup pure maple syrup

INSTRUCTIONS:

Combine the oat milk, cayenne pepper to taste, Dijon mustard, and maple syrup in a bowl, stir well, and serve.

RASPBERRY SALAD DRESSING

My mom has a thing for raspberries. We can always find them in her fridge or freezer—fresh or frozen, she works them into her day. We think this dressing is delicious, even by the spoonful. Try it on a mesclun mix with orange slices.

INGREDIENTS:

- 1 cup fresh or frozen raspberries (defrosted, if frozen)
- ¼ cup apple cider vinegar or white balsamic vinegar
- 2 cloves garlic, minced
- 1 tablespoon Dijon mustard
- 6 to 8 red grapes
- ⅛ teaspoon freshly ground black pepper

INSTRUCTIONS:

In a food processor, combine the raspberries, apple cider vinegar, garlic, Dijon mustard, grapes, and pepper. Process until smooth. Serve on salads or greens or even desserts!

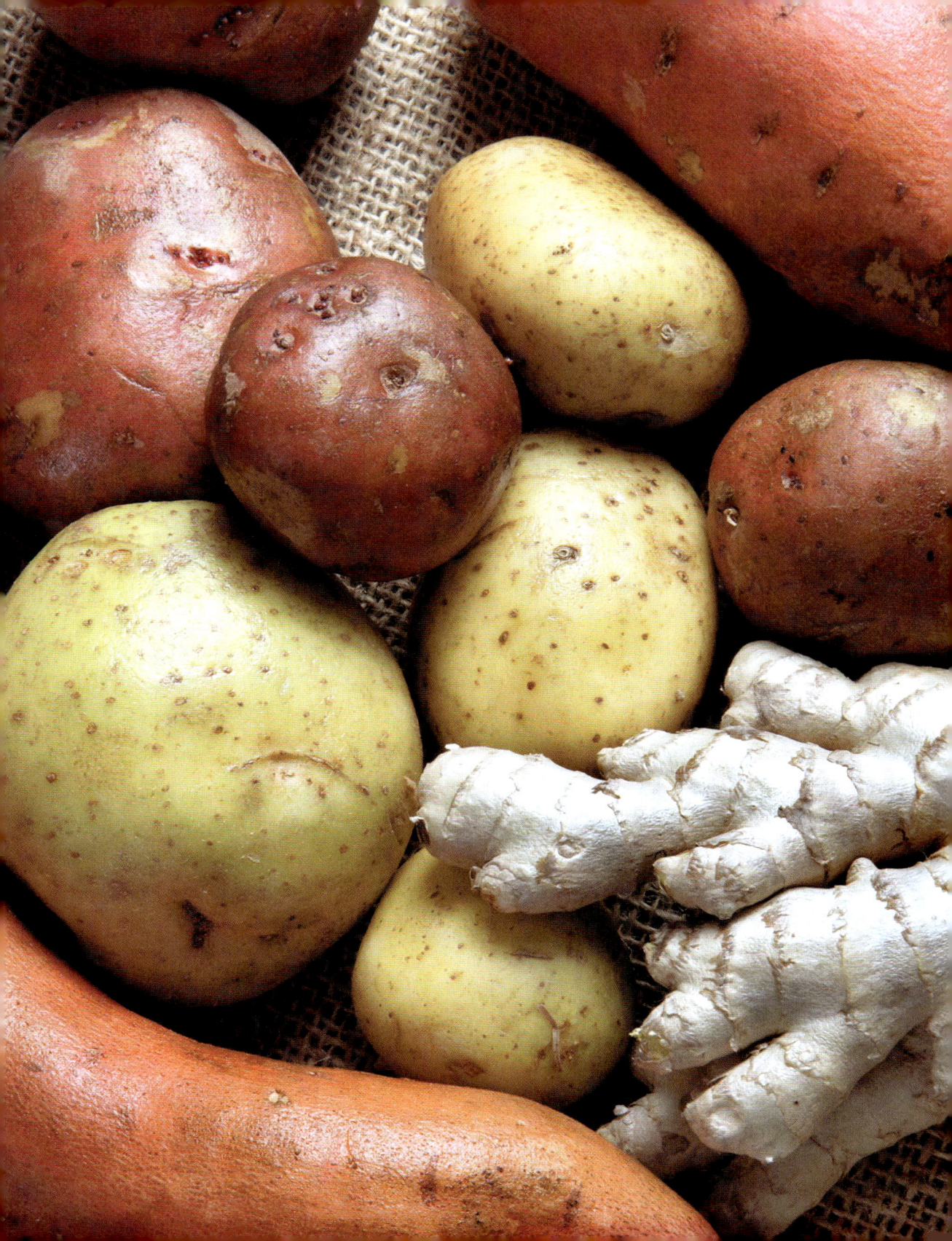

DINNERS

Now it's time for the main event. But here's a secret: The main dish for any meal can be as simple as a baked sweet or white potato with some fabulous, hearty vegetable sides or salads. It could even be a few ears of fabulous farm-fresh corn when it's in season along with Jen's Potato Salad with Fresh Dill (page 139). We rarely fuss over more than one part of a meal.

Our favorite go-to, one-bowl hearty meal is rice and beans, and we include our favorite recipe here. But you may crave more complex dinners some nights or want a special meal to wow guests (though all our guests love our rice and beans!). There is nothing more fun—when you have time—than making something that looks impressive and tastes delicious. So try it all! Here are our lasagnas, slow-cook bean dishes, pizzas, pastas, burritos, dals, burgers, stuffed portobellos, and many more. Tweak things by adding your own touch with favorite ingredients or eliminating things you don't like. But always include those greens!

Most important, remember you can eat well and eat simply. If you find something you like, eat it often. Get into a pattern. There is no magic in variety. The magic is in discovering what eating a whole-food, plant-based diet with *no oil added* does for you.

TRIPLE-DECKER LASAGNA

Nothing is more satisfying than lasagna. This dish is tall, hearty, colorful, and delish! It's three layers of plant-based filling and three layers of noodles, like a triple-decker bunk bed. Go ahead and follow our directions the first time, and next time play around, if you'd like, and change what filling goes where. Or create new layers of plant-based filling! This lasagna would be terrific with eggplant, kale, broccoli, peppers—oh, the endless possibilities! A great dish to prepare ahead—as it is good the next day, or arguably even better *the next day!*

INGREDIENTS:

1 large onion, diced (2 to 3 cups)

2 cloves garlic, minced

2 medium zucchini, sliced (2 to 3 cups)

1 medium yellow squash, sliced (2 to 3 cups)

16 ounces mushrooms, sliced

8 ounces frozen spinach, thawed

2 cups Napa cabbage, sliced

1 tablespoon dried thyme

1 tablespoon dried oregano

1 teaspoon garlic powder

3 sweet potatoes, cooked, peeled, and mashed (about 3 cups mashed)

¼ teaspoon grated nutmeg

3 or 4 (25-ounce) jars of no-oil-added pasta sauce (some of us like more sauce than
    others) or 8 to 9 cups Light and Easy Marinara (page 125)

2 boxes whole wheat lasagna noodles, uncooked

3 to 4 Roma tomatoes, sliced

½ cup nutritional yeast

Preheat the oven to 350°F.

In a frying pan, cook the onions and garlic over high heat, stirring continuously, until the onions turn soft and translucent. Add water if the pan gets too dry. Reduce the heat to medium-high and add the zucchini, yellow squash, mushrooms, spinach, cabbage, thyme, and oregano, and cook until cooked through. Set aside.

In a bowl, combine the mashed sweet potato and nutmeg, and mix until smooth and uniform in color and texture.

To construct the lasagna, in the base of a lasagna pan, pour a layer of pasta sauce, then add a layer of noodles. Atop the noodles add a layer of cooked vegetables (use exactly half of the vegetable mixture from the pan), and then add another layer of red sauce. On top of the red sauce place a layer of noodles, and then a layer of sweet potato. On top of the sweet potato add a layer of sauce and another layer of noodles. Then add another layer of cooked vegetables (the other half from the pan) and a layer of red sauce. Then add the last layer of noodles, and top it off with a layer of sauce. In a nice pattern, lay the tomato slices on top of the red sauce so they cover the whole surface. Finally, sprinkle a thick layer of nutritional yeast over the entire top.

Cover with foil and bake for 45 minutes. Remove the foil and bake for 15 minutes more while the top layer browns.

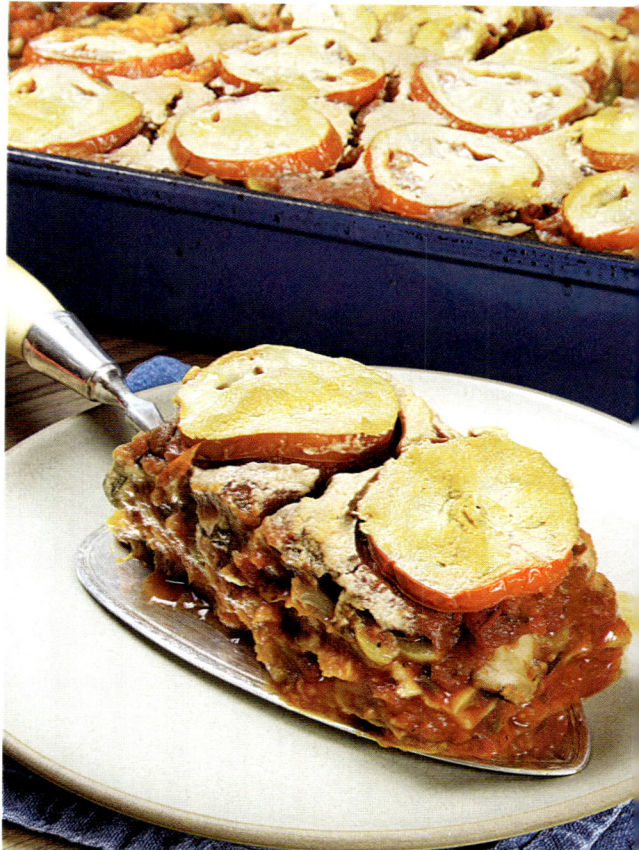

EAT LOAF

We all love this dish. It is just like meat loaf—thus the name "Eat Loaf." I had a large pot of white beans and a refrigerator full of greens to use up when I created the recipe for this loaf. It is irresistible sliced with steamed vegetables and a salad, or on a whole-grain bun or bread with lettuce and tomato (beware—it squishes), or "fried" in a nonstick pan with no oil the next day for lunch or dinner.

INGREDIENTS:

1 large onion, chopped

3 large cloves garlic, minced

8 ounces mushrooms, sliced

½ jalapeño, seeded and diced

2 cups diced zucchini

½ cup shredded carrots

½ red bell pepper, seeded and diced

1 tomato, cored and diced

4 cups spinach or greens of your choice like Swiss chard, collards, or kale

½ cup chopped fresh cilantro or parsley

½ teaspoon freshly ground black pepper, or to taste

½ teaspoon freshly ground white pepper, or to taste

1 teaspoon Mrs. Dash seasoning mix or other no-salt seasoning

2 (15-ounce) cans no-salt-added cannellini or navy beans, drained and rinsed

2 cups old-fashioned oats

½ cup prepared salsa

1 cup barbecue sauce or ketchup (find a brand with no high-fructose corn syrup)

INSTRUCTIONS:

Preheat the oven to 350°F.

In a nonstick frying pan, cook the onions for a few minutes over medium-high heat until they begin to soften. Add water if the pan gets too dry. Add the garlic, mushrooms, jalapeño, zucchini, carrots, bell pepper, and tomatoes, and keep cooking for 5 to 8 minutes, or until the zucchini is soft.

Add the spinach to the vegetable mixture and continue cooking until the greens are wilted and soft. (Swiss chard softens quickly. Kale or collards take a few minutes longer to wilt and soften.)

Add the cilantro, black pepper, white pepper, and Mrs. Dash, and stir.

In a medium bowl, combine the beans, oats, and salsa. Add the vegetable mixture and stir. Use your hands here if needed to mix everything well and to mash some of the beans. When it becomes sort of sticky (mortar-like), it is ready for the loaf pans.

Coat the bottom of two loaf pans with ¼ cup (or less) each of barbecue sauce and add half of the vegetable-bean mixture to each pan. On top of the vegetable-bean mixture, spread another layer of barbecue sauce.

Bake for 1 hour. Let cool a bit before cutting into the "eat" loaf. It cuts *much* better when it has had time to cool and set.

Serve warm, with greens and smiles!

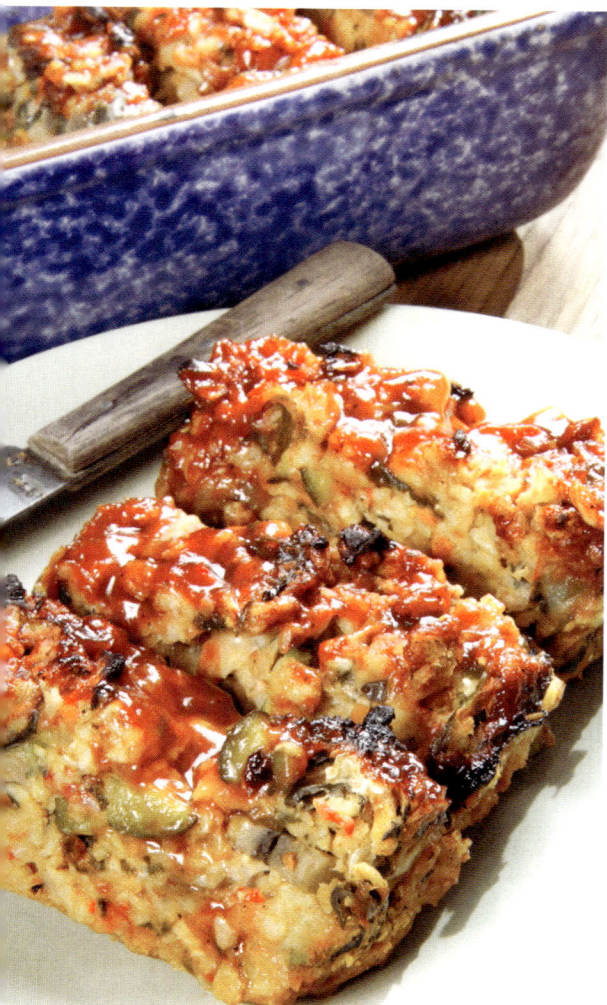

TRIPLE PEPPER-CROWNED RISOTTO

I made this dish right around the time a racehorse was poised to win the Triple Crown. The horse did not end up winning, but this savory, colorful dish did! The three beautiful peppers looked so royal atop the risotto—Triple Pepper–Crowned Risotto.

INGREDIENTS:

2 cups short-grain brown rice (short-grain is preferred as it gets stickier)

4 cups vegetable broth

1 onion, diced

3 to 4 cloves garlic, minced

8 ounces mushrooms, sliced

3 to 4 cups kale, stems removed and leaves torn into pieces and cooked

Roasted Red Peppers (page 24)—follow the recipe using red bell peppers, yellow bell peppers, and orange bell peppers

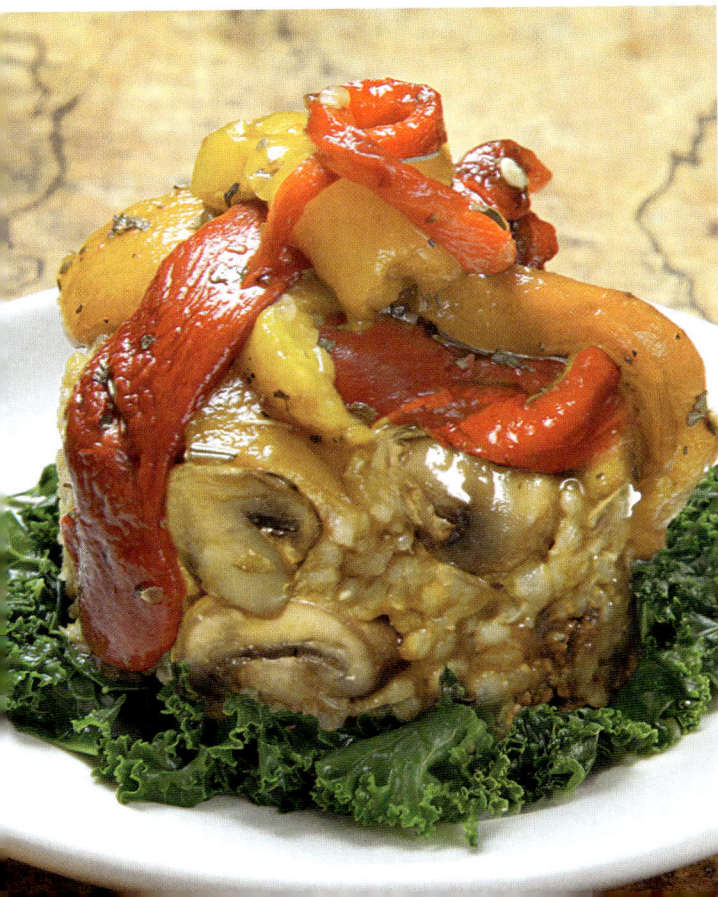

INSTRUCTIONS:

In a rice cooker or on the stovetop, prepare the rice as directed using the broth (not water) and adding the onions, garlic, and mushrooms.

Stir the warm rice for a minute or so until it uniformly becomes a bit creamier and stickier—it is now called risotto. Using small bowls or teacups as molds, scoop about ½ cup of risotto to make the number of servings you desire. These molds create nice, thronelike shapes for the peppers to handsomely rest upon when served.

To serve, arrange a bed of cooked kale on a plate, flip a bowl or cup of the risotto upside down onto the kale. Crown the risotto with the luscious peppers. Serve with a salad, and heaps of broccoli, and eat like kings!

RED THAI CURRY VEGGIES OVER
BROWN BASMATI RICE

I love Thai food, especially all different types of curry. When I learned what was in a Thai curry—spices mixed with coconut milk—I did not fret. There is a plant-based answer to avoiding all the saturated fat in coconut milk: coconut extract plus nondairy milk. Ta-da—coconut milk, or as we call it "faux-conut" milk! Coconut lovers will never know the difference. But your body will.

INGREDIENTS:

8 ounces mushrooms, sliced

1 large onion, sliced

2 heads broccoli, cut into florets

1 red bell pepper, diced

2 carrots, sliced into thin rounds

2 cups plain unsweetened oat milk

1 teaspoon coconut extract

1 tablespoon maple syrup

2 to 3 teaspoons green or red curry paste (Thai Kitchen makes an oil-free variety)

2 cups brown basmati rice, cooked as directed on the package

6 to 8 leaves Thai basil, finely chopped

INSTRUCTIONS:

In a large frying pan, cook the mushrooms and onions over high heat, gradually reducing the heat as they brown. Add the broccoli, bell pepper, and carrots, cover, and cook until their colors turn bright and they still have snap, about 5 minutes.

In a saucepan over medium-high heat, combine the oat milk, coconut extract, maple syrup, and curry paste. Stir until warm and well combined. Pour over the cooked vegetables, and serve over cooked brown basmati rice with a garnish of Thai basil on top and, of course, a salad of kale on the side.

ROASTED ROOTS

On a rainy fall day in Cleveland, Ohio, nothing smells better that the aroma of roasting roots. They take a while to cook, so there is plenty of time to run errands, nap, or make a cornucopia of other dishes! The key here is to go for it*! Try including any root vegetables: beets, sweet potatoes, parsnips, turnips, rutabaga, horseradish root, celery root, or any other gnarly roots. Be sure to serve this with a heaping salad and Cooked Kale (page 23).*

INGREDIENTS:

- 1 large onion, diced
- 2 Yukon Gold potatoes, diced (about 3 cups)
- 1 large or 2 small sweet potatoes, diced (about 3 cups)
- 1 turnip, peeled and diced (about 1 cup)
- 1 cup diced rutabaga, wax coating removed
- 1 parsnip, peeled and diced (optional)
- 1 celery root, peeled and diced (optional)
- 2 beets, peeled and diced (optional)
- 1 teaspoon dried thyme
- 1 teaspoon dried rosemary
- ½ teaspoon minced garlic

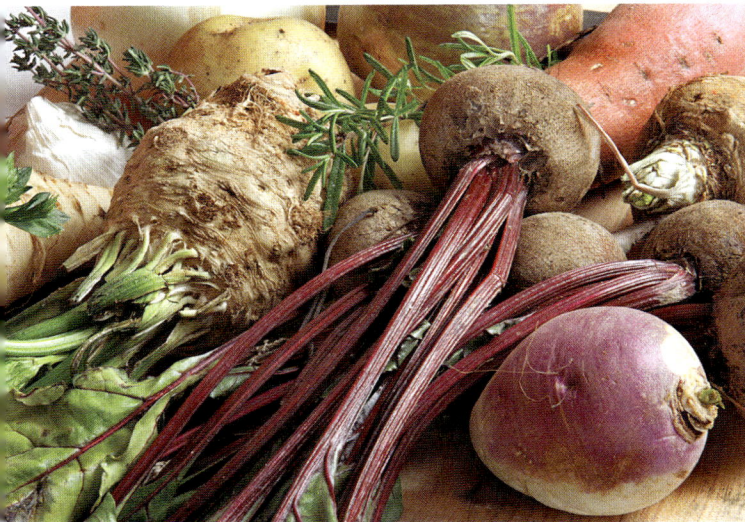

INSTRUCTIONS:

Preheat the oven to 350°F.

In a roasting pan or lasagna pan, place the onions, potatoes, sweet potato, turnip, rutabaga, and optional root vegetables of your choice. Add the thyme, rosemary, and garlic, and toss. Cover the pan with foil and cook for 1 hour.

Serve warm with a huge salad and steamed greens.

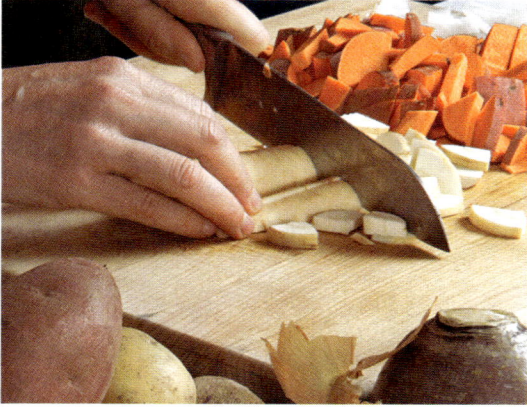
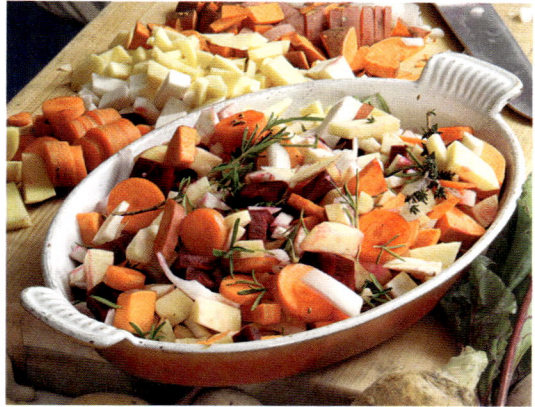
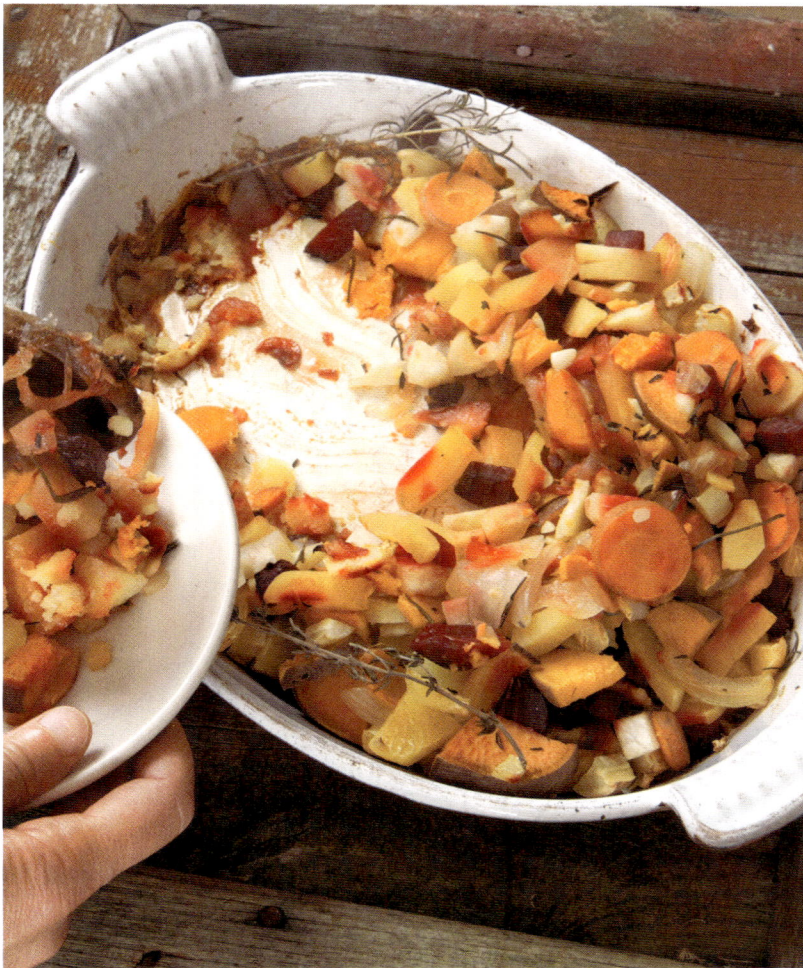

PACIFIC RIM SOBA NOODLES

Soba noodles—warm or cold—are a family favorite! This recipe makes a great warm dinner one night and a filling cold lunch the next day. It is also our summer go-to meal when guests arrive. And, of course, serving these soba noodles over a bed of collard greens keeps our endothelial cells happily regenerating!

INGREDIENTS:

4 cups collard greens, stems removed, leaves cut into long, thin ½-inch strips

16 ounces buckwheat or whole wheat soba noodles, cooked as directed on the package

1 red bell pepper, cubed

2 to 3 green onions, chopped

1 mango, cubed

⅓ cup shredded carrots

1 tablespoon minced peeled fresh ginger

6 tablespoons low-sodium tamari, or less, to taste

¼ cup pure maple syrup

3 tablespoons rice vinegar

INSTRUCTIONS:

Bring an inch or two of water to boil in a saucepan and cook the collard strips until dark green and softened. Drain and set aside.

In a large bowl, combine the cooked soba noodles, bell peppers, green onions, mango, and carrots, and toss.

In a small bowl, combine the ginger, tamari, maple syrup, and rice vinegar. Stir until uniformly mixed, and then pour over the noodle mixture. To serve, place a handful of the cooked collard green strips in the base of each bowl and then add dressed soba noodles. Toss and eat!

KALE-STUFFED TUGBOATS

These stuffed potatoes are mighty favorites, not to mention how adorable and delectable they are! They will fill you up and keep you tugging and chugging along for hours. Make more than you think you will need. They are a fantastic lunch the next day, if they last until then!

INGREDIENTS:

6 medium Yukon Gold potatoes

1 large sweet onion

2 cloves garlic

1 bunch kale, stems stripped and leaves chopped

2 teaspoons onion powder

2 teaspoons garlic powder

1 tablespoon balsamic vinegar

Pinch of cayenne pepper

½ to 1 teaspoon freshly ground black pepper

6 tablespoons nutritional yeast

½ to 1 cup unsweetened almond milk

3 green onions, chopped

2 cups frozen corn

½ red bell pepper, diced (about ½ cup)

Paprika, regular or smoked, for dusting

INSTRUCTIONS:

Preheat the oven to 450°F.

Scrub the potatoes and pierce them in a few spots with a knife. Remove the outside skin from the onion, chop roughly, and wrap the onion in foil. Slip the garlic cloves into the foil, too.

Bake the wrapped onion and garlic and the potatoes for 1 hour. Remove from the oven, and reduce the oven temperature to 350°F.

Place the baked onion and garlic in a food processor and blend until liquid. This will work, as most of your liquid is in the potatoes.

Bring a pot of water to a boil and cook the kale for about 5 minutes, or until tender. Drain the kale, and set aside.

Cut the potatoes in half, scoop out their flesh, place it in a medium bowl, and mash with a potato masher or fork until crumbly. Arrange the empty potato skins in a baking dish.

Add the onion puree to the potatoes along with the onion powder, garlic powder, balsamic vinegar, cayenne, black pepper, nutritional yeast, and almond milk, and mix well. Add more liquid if needed to achieve the consistency of mashed potatoes. If the onion is large you may just need ½ cup of almond milk (or none).

Gently stir in the green onions, corn, and bell peppers. Finally, carefully incorporate the kale.

Fill each skin to heaping with the potato and vegetable mixture.

Sprinkle with paprika and bake for 30 minutes or until beginning to brown.

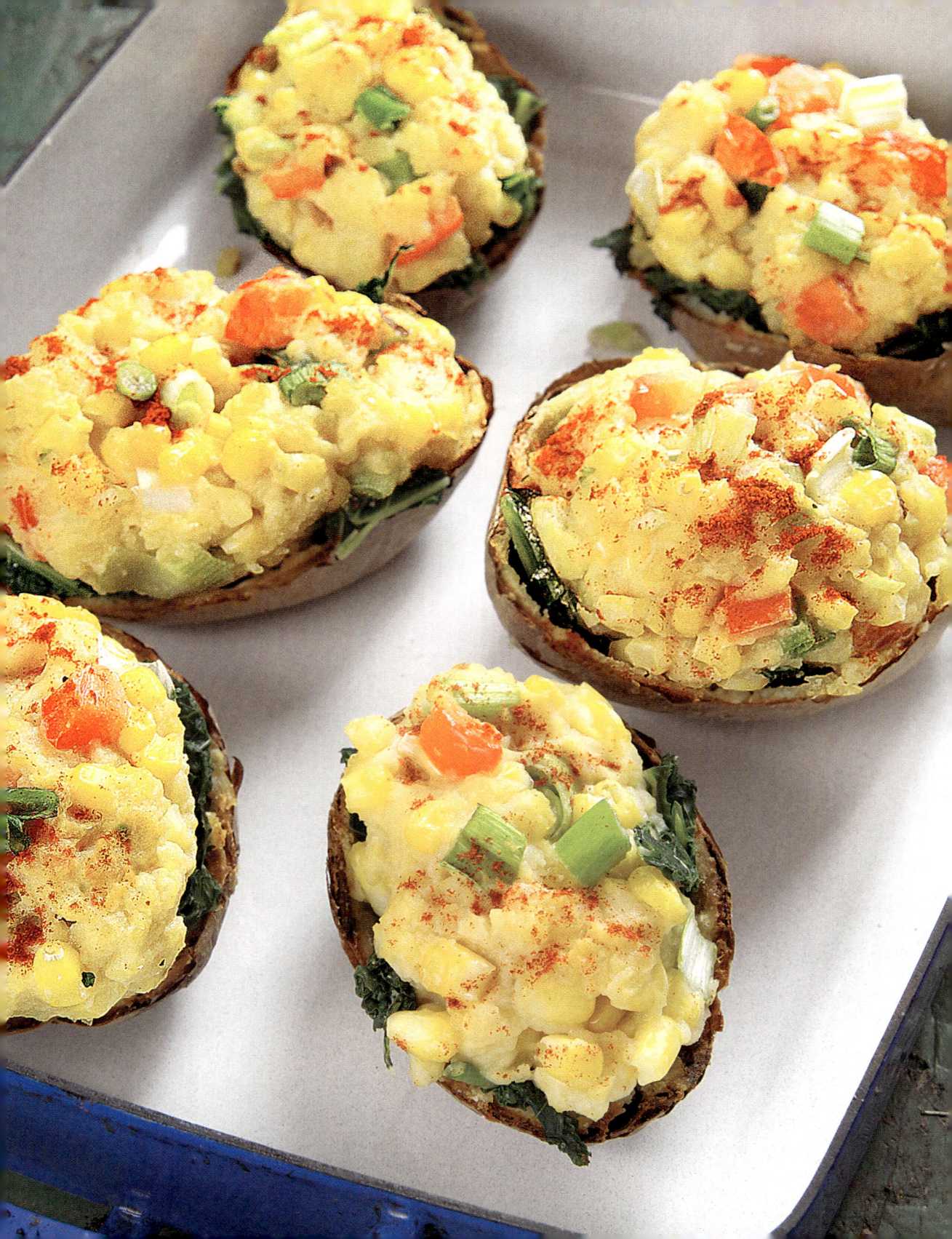

SANDRA'S CHILI

Our son Zeb invited his graduating Columbia School of Journalism class for an evening at the farm where we spend time in the summer. In a pot about three feet tall, over an outdoor fire, Sandra, a fellow student, made a chili everyone loved. And it was also beautiful looking. Below is the recipe inspired by Sandra's creation—with ingredients to serve eight, not eighty! Sandra wondered what to use instead of oil to cook the onions and settled on beer. That is a choice up to you, but any liquid will work. The flavors bloom the longer the chili cooks, so don't worry if you make this a day or two ahead of time—it will taste even better. We like to serve this scooped into Corn Tortilla Taco Shells and Tostados (page 32) or in Crispy Tortilla Bowls (page 30).

INGREDIENTS:

- 1 large onion, chopped
- 3 carrots, chopped
- 4 stalks celery, chopped
- 1 large red bell pepper, seeded and chopped
- 1 medium zucchini, chopped
- 1 jalapeño, seeded and chopped
- 4 cloves garlic, chopped
- 8 ounces mushrooms, sliced
- 1 (28-ounce) can whole tomatoes
- 1 (15-ounce) can diced tomatoes
- 1 (15-ounce) can no-salt-added dark red kidney beans, drained and rinsed
- 1 (15-ounce) can no-salt-added chickpeas, drained and rinsed
- 1 (15-ounce) can no-salt-added black beans, drained and rinsed
- 1 large sweet potato, peeled, if desired, and diced
- 1 teaspoon dried thyme
- 3 tablespoons chili powder, plus more as needed
- 1 teaspoon ground cumin
- 1 cup salsa, your favorite
- Freshly ground black pepper
- 2 tablespoons balsamic vinegar
- Cooked brown rice or barley, for serving
- ½ cup sliced green onions

In a large soup pot, cook the onions over medium-high heat until just starting to soften. Add liquid (water—or beer!) as necessary if the bottom gets dry.

Add the carrots and continue cooking for a few minutes. Then add the celery, stir, and cook for 1 minute more. Reduce the heat to medium, add the bell pepper, zucchini, jalapeño, garlic, and mushrooms, and cook, stirring, until the vegetables begin to wilt.

Add the whole tomatoes, diced tomatoes, kidney beans, chickpeas, black beans, sweet potato, thyme, chili, and cumin. Bring to a boil; then reduce heat to maintain a simmer. Cover the chili while it simmers for 1 hour, or until it has thickened and all vegetables are soft. Add salsa, pepper, and balsmic vinegar, and stir.

Serve over rice or barley in huge bowls sprinkled with green onions, alongside a great salad.

TORTILLA AZTECA-MEXICAN LASAGNA

Our friend Norma treated us to nearly ten recipes from her home in Mexico. Her grandmother from Toluca, Mexico, used to make this dish in winter with vegetables she had on hand. Norma made this for us in December with the vegetables from the grocery store but also with some of the greens from our garden. (True! Greens grow in December in Cleveland.) This dish rings with authenticity and flavors from Mexico. We loved it and bet you will love it, too. Thank you, Norma!

INGREDIENTS:

1 large sweet onion, julienned

4 poblano peppers, seeded and cut into thin strips

2 medium zucchini, julienned or cut into matchsticks

16 ounces frozen or fresh corn

8 ounces mushrooms, sliced

2 (15-ounce) cans no-salt-added pinto beans, drained and rinsed

1 cup vegetable broth or water

2 large tomatoes, roughly chopped

¼ onion, diced

1 large clove garlic, minced

1 green chile (also called a finger chile), seeded

10 corn tortillas

1 cup Enchilada Sauce (page 114)

1 to 2 cups salsa, your favorite

1 Anaheim pepper, sliced into thin rounds

INSTRUCTIONS:

Preheat the oven to 400°F.

In a large frying pan, cook the julienned onions over high heat, gradually reducing the heat as the onions get limp and brown. Add the poblano peppers and continue to cook, stirring, for another minute. Add the zucchini, corn, and mushrooms, and cook on low for 10 minutes, or until everything is soft.

Place half of the pinto beans and the vegetable broth in a blender or food processor and blend until it is souplike. Pour the bean mixture into a small bowl.

Place the tomatoes, diced onions, garlic, and seeded green chile in a food processor, and process until smooth. Pour this mixture into a saucepan and cook on medium heat for 5 minutes, until warmed through and the color has changed from orange to red. This is called a Tortilla Azteca sauce.

In the bottom of a large casserole pan, spread a layer of the Tortilla Azteca sauce. On top of the sauce, arrange a layer of tortillas so that none of the sauce below shows through. If needed, tear some tortillas into pieces and patch exposed areas. On top of the tortillas, add the cooked vegetables. Cover the vegetables with the blended bean mixture, and on top of the bean mixture, add a layer of the remaining whole pinto beans.

Add another complete layer of tortillas (no beans showing through from below) on top of the beans. On top of the tortillas, add a layer of Enchilada Sauce and a layer of salsa.

We like to top it all off with decoratively placed, thinly sliced rounds of Anaheim pepper. The green and red contrast is beautiful.

Bake for 30 minutes. Do not overcook. Serve hot.

TOMATO CHUTNEY OVER CARAMELIZED ONION HUMMUS PIZZA

MAKES 1 (12-INCH) PIZZA; SERVES 2 TO 4

Debbie Kastner, author of the Happy Healthy Long Life *blog, shared a version of this with us and we loved how beautiful and tasty it was! In fact, we even wanted this pizza on the cover of the book. We've found some terrific, no-oil pizza crusts: Sami's Millet and Flax Pizza Crust (Samisbakery.com), Nature's Hilights Brown Rice Pizza Crust, and Whole Foods whole wheat dough, for example. You can also make this pizza with whole wheat pita bread or make your own dough (without any oil). Serve this beautiful pizza with a heaping salad of greens!*

INGREDIENTS:

1 (12-inch) Sami's Millet and Flax Pizza Crust, or similar

1½ cups Caramelized Onion Hummus (page 104)

2 cups Cherry Tomato Chutney (page 108)

INSTRUCTIONS:

Preheat the oven to 350°F.

Bake the pizza crust (without the toppings) for 10 minutes, until golden brown but not too crisp. Spread the pizza crust with a nice thick layer of the Caramelized Onion Hummus. Spread the Cherry Tomato Chutney evenly on top of the hummus. It is such a beautiful pizza, so snap a photo, slice, and serve!

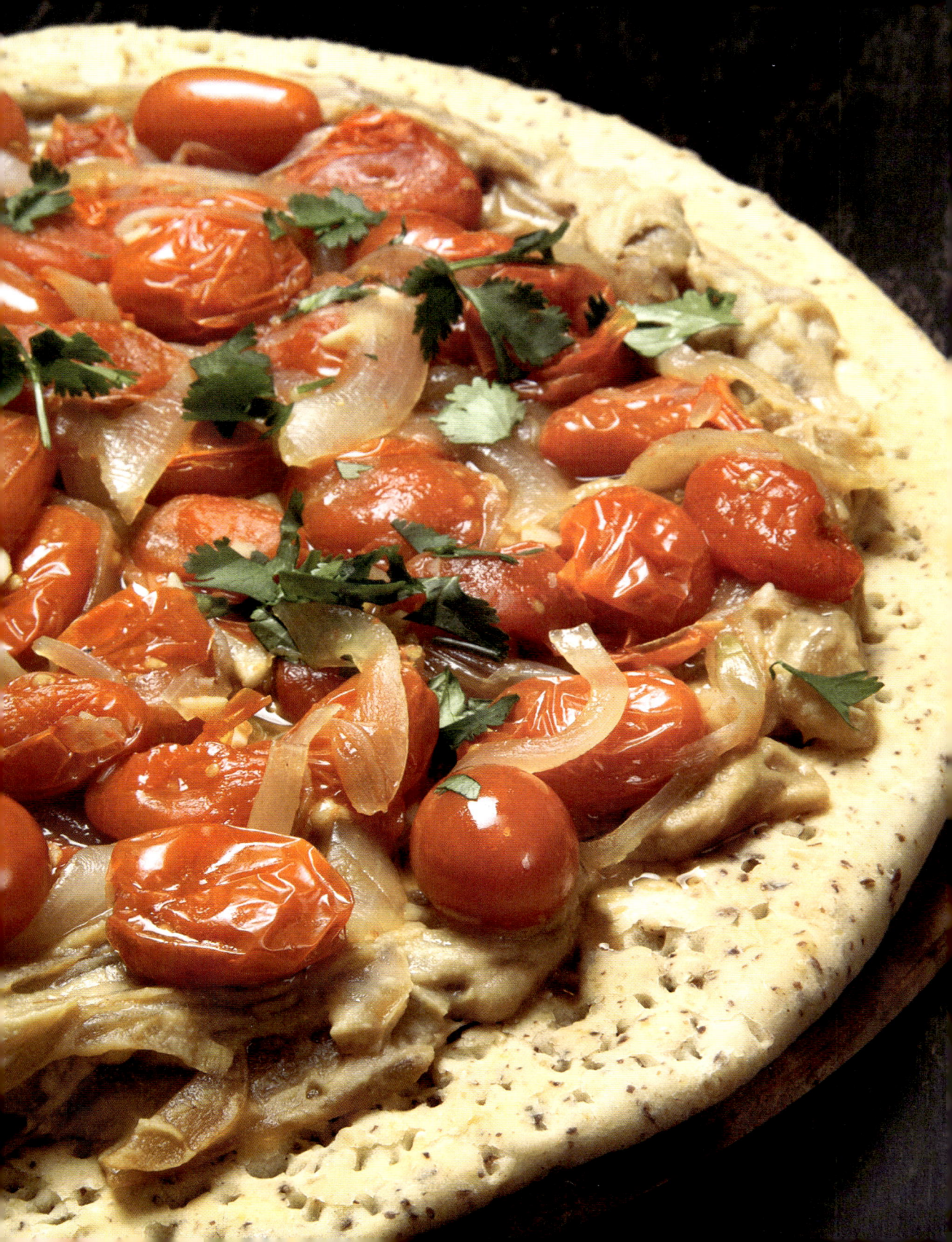

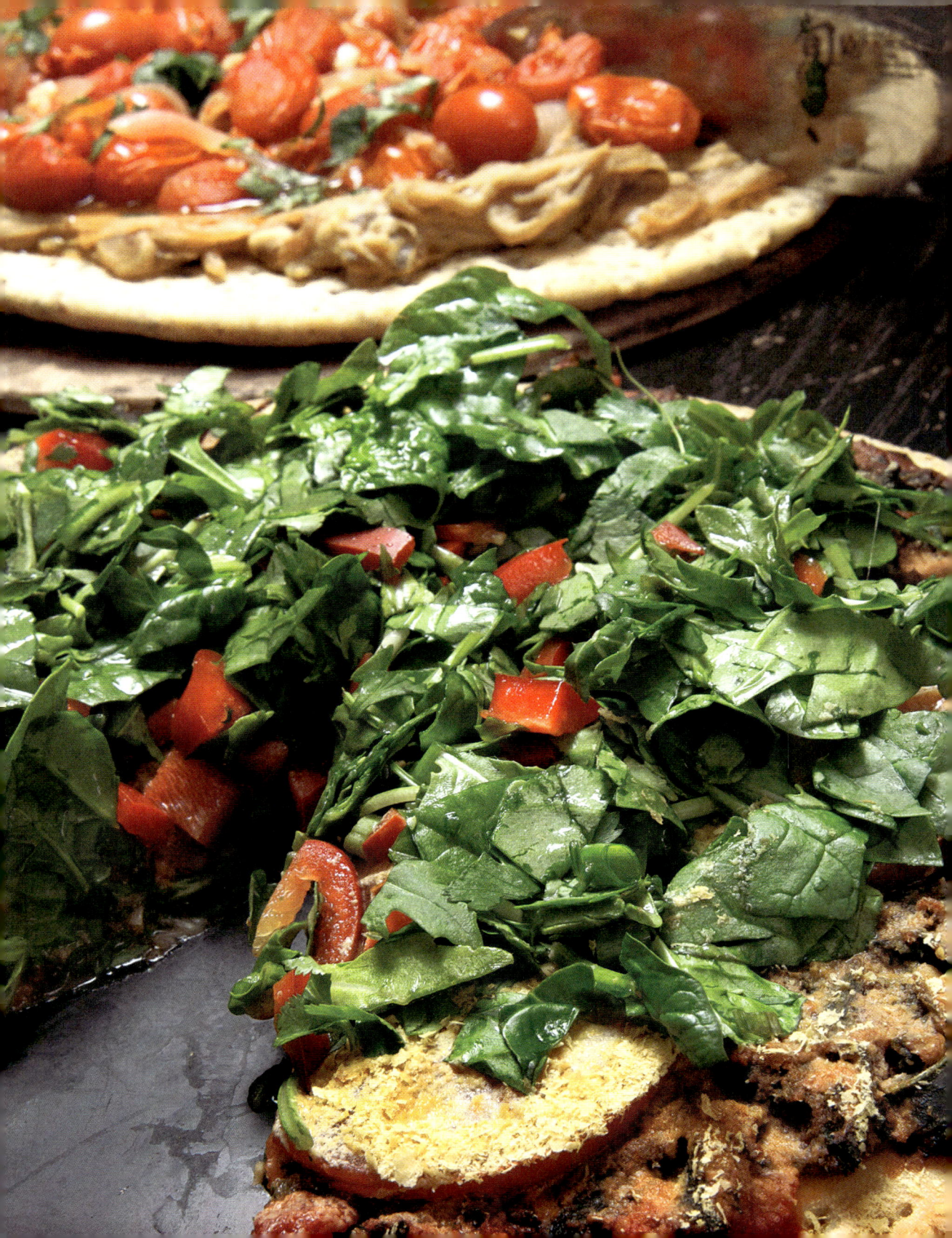

SALAD PIZZA

Charlene, one of the most enthusiastic plant-based eaters we know, sent us the idea for this pizza with salad on top! She said this is how they are serving it in Italy now! The fun thing is that anything in the refrigerator will work on top. We add chopped greens in with our pizza sauce as an easy way to get more greens on board. Be innovative. Again, you can make your own dough or try Sami's, Nature's Hilights Brown Rice Pizza Crust, or Whole Foods whole wheat dough. Whole wheat pita bread also works. Sami's Millet and Flax Pizza Crust is our favorite and it is available online. It is absolutely delicious and worth hunting down at samisbakery.com.

INGREDIENTS:

1½ to 2 cups no-oil-added pasta sauce

1 cup Cooked Kale (page 23), collards, or Swiss chard

1 (12-inch) Sami's Millet and Flax Pizza Crust, or similar

3 to 4 tomatoes, sliced thinly

3 to 4 tablespoons nutritional yeast

2 cups spinach, chopped

2 cups arugula, chopped

2 green onions, chopped

¼ cup basil, chopped

1 red bell pepper, chopped

1 to 2 tablespoons fresh lemon juice

INSTRUCTIONS:

Preheat the oven to 450°F.

Mix the pasta sauce with the Cooked Kale, and spread it out evenly on the pizza crust.

Arrange the tomato slices over the sauce. Sprinkle the tomatoes with nutritional yeast and place the pizza in the oven for 20 minutes.

In a bowl, make a salad out of the spinach, arugula, green onions, basil, and bell pepper. Sprinkle the salad with lemon juice and toss well.

Remove the pizza from the oven and heap the salad on top of it.

Slice this beauty with a pizza cutter and serve up one big slice of yum!

ASPARAGUS MUSHROOM PIE WITH LEMONY CHEEZY SAUCE

SERVES 3 TO 4

This is fun to make and even more fun to eat! It helps to use short-grain brown rice for the crust as it sticks together better. The pie will cut into wedgelike heaps better if it cools a little before you cut it, but it is just as good in messy little heaps. Sweet Corn Sauce (page 111) is also a good variation for a topping.

INGREDIENTS:

2 cups cooked short-grain brown rice

1 teaspoon garlic powder

3 teaspoons Mrs. Dash lemon pepper, divided

1 large tomato, sliced thinly, or ½ pint cherry tomatoes, halved

4 green onions, chopped (½ cup)

8 ounces mushrooms, sliced

2 tablespoons balsamic vinegar

1 bunch asparagus, trimmed and cut in 1-inch pieces (about 2 cups)

I bunch kale, stems stripped and leaves chopped into pieces

1½ cups Lemony Cheezy Sauce (page 112)

2 tablespoons nutritional yeast

INSTRUCTIONS:

Preheat the oven to 350°F.

Place the rice in a large bowl, add the garlic powder and 2 teaspoons of the lemon pepper, and mix well with a fork.

In an 8-inch pie plate, spread rice evenly along the bottom and up the sides.

Arrange the tomato slices on the rice, and then sprinkle the tomatoes with half the chopped green onions.

In a frying pan, lay the mushrooms flat (totally flat) on the surface of the pan, and cook over medium heat for 5 minutes without turning. Sprinkle the mushrooms with 1 tablespoon of the balsamic vinegar, stir, and cook for another minute, until the mushrooms have browned. Place the mushrooms and any of their juice over the tomatoes.

Add the asparagus to the pan and cook for 4 to 5 minutes, until bright green and tender.

Add liquid as necessary. Drain and run the asparagus briefly under cold water to stop the cooking. Arrange the asparagus on top of the mushrooms and sprinkle with the remaining 1 teaspoon lemon pepper and about 2 tablespoons of the green onions, saving a few of the green onions for the top.

Cook the kale in 2 inches of boiling water for 4 to 5 minutes; then drain and squeeze out any extra water. Arrange the kale over the asparagus and sprinkle with the remaining 1 tablespoon of balsamic vinegar.

Spread the Lemony Cheezy Sauce over the surface of the pie, sprinkle with the last few green onions and nutritional yeast, and bake for 30 minutes.

Allow the pie to cool for 10 minutes before serving—there's a greater chance the pie wedges will hold their shape. If not, enjoy the messy heaps!

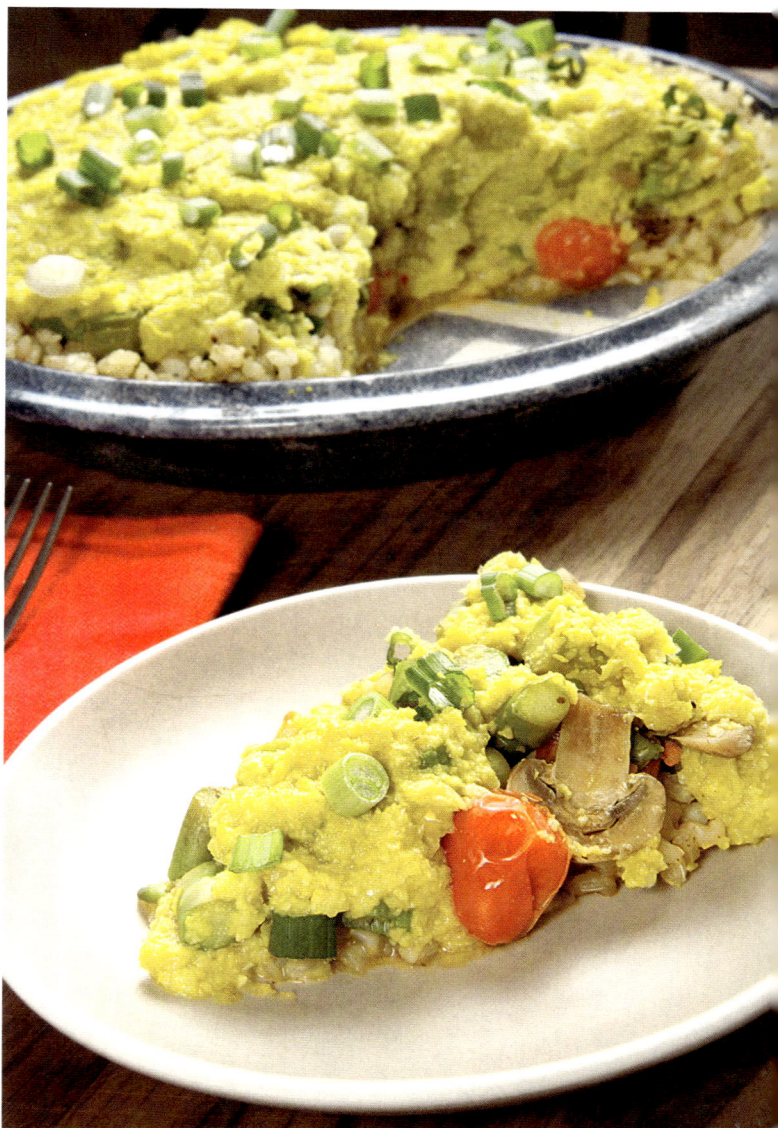

POLENTA PIE

Polenta was not a favorite until Rip made us a polenta pie. We licked the platter clean. This easy-to-assemble pie is one we often serve, and it is oh so filling!

INGREDIENTS:

1 cup cornmeal

½ teaspoon garlic powder

½ teaspoon onion powder

1½ teaspoons ground cumin, divided

Pinch of cayenne pepper

2 cups fresh spinach

1 (15-ounce) can no-salt-added pinto beans, drained and rinsed

1 medium onion, diced

1 red bell pepper, diced

1 cup frozen roasted corn, thawed

1 teaspoon chili powder

2 teaspoons Tex-Mex seasoning or taco seasoning, your choice (look for no added oils), or see Tip on the following page

2 ounces green chiles, diced (optional)

½ fresh jalapeño pepper, seeded and diced (optional)

½ cup Enchilada Sauce (page 114; optional)

½ cup salsa, your favorite brand

INSTRUCTIONS:

Preheat the oven to 400°F. Line a 9-inch pie pan with parchment paper.

Bring 3 cups water to a boil in a large saucepan. While whisking continuously, slowly add in the cornmeal and reduce the heat to low. Keep stirring until all the lumps are gone. Add the garlic powder, onion powder, ½ teaspoon of the cumin, and the cayenne, and stir until the polenta is thick and has no lumps at all, about 15 minutes.

Shape the polenta into the lined pie pan using the back of a spoon or your fingers. It should be about ¼ to ½ inch thick all over.

Into the newly formed polenta piecrust add the fresh spinach as the bottom layer. On top of the spinach add the pinto beans.

In a bowl, combine the onions, bell peppers, corn, chili powder, Tex-Mex seasoning, remaining 1 teaspoon of cumin, green chiles (if using), and jalapeño (if using), and toss.

On top of the pinto beans, add the vegetable filling from the bowl. On top of it all pour and spread Enchilada Sauce (if using) and salsa.

Bake for 50 minutes. Serve warm with more salsa, Enchilada Sauce, if desired, and a heaping salad and greens alongside!

TIP:

To make your own Tex-Mex seasoning, just combine the dry spices from our Tex-Mex Kale Chips recipe (page 143)!

FIVE-STAR RICE AND BEANS

SERVES 8 TO 10

This is the meal we eat most of all. This is the meal that we serve when guests come over. This is the meal we have on Christmas Eve. We have served it at weddings and even at our fiftieth wedding anniversary. This is what a great deal of the world eats a great deal of the time. For us, it is all about the toppings—all about the toppings! Our grandchildren like to fill Corn Tortilla Taco Shells (page 32) with all of the fillings and fixings.

INGREDIENTS:

5 (15-ounce) cans no-salt-added black beans, drained and rinsed

1 tablespoon ground cumin

2 teaspoons onion powder

1 tablespoon garlic powder

2 tablespoons chili powder

¼ teaspoon cayenne pepper

½ cup salsa, your favorite

10 Corn Tortilla Taco Shells (page 32)

4 cups brown rice, cooked according to the package directions

12 ounces frozen corn, thawed

1 red bell pepper, seeded and cubed

1 yellow bell pepper, seeded and cubed

1 orange bell pepper, seeded and cubed

3 cups kale, stems stripped and leaves chopped into bite-size pieces and cooked

3 large tomatoes, cored and cubed

1 bunch green onions, chopped

8 ounces water chestnuts, sliced

1 cup shredded carrots

1 small jicama, peeled and diced

2 cups fresh cilantro, chopped

Lots of different salsas: Mango-Lime Salsa (page 120), Pico de Gallo (page 119), Down Under Cranberry Salsa (page 121), Pomegranate Salsa (page 124), or other salsas of your choice

Place the black beans in a large skillet over medium heat. Add the cumin, onion powder, garlic powder, chili powder, and cayenne, and stir. Add the ½ cup salsa to the bean mixture if you feel it needs moisture and flavor. Taste and tweak it to your preference. Use an immersion blender or fork to blend or smash up half of the beans.

To serve, set up a buffet so it flows from rice and beans to all the veggies. We set up our buffet bowls in the following order: brown rice, black beans, tomatoes, corn, peppers, kale, green onions, water chestnuts, carrots, jicama, cilantro, and the variety of salsas.

Everyone makes his or her own colorful, delicious mountain of food.

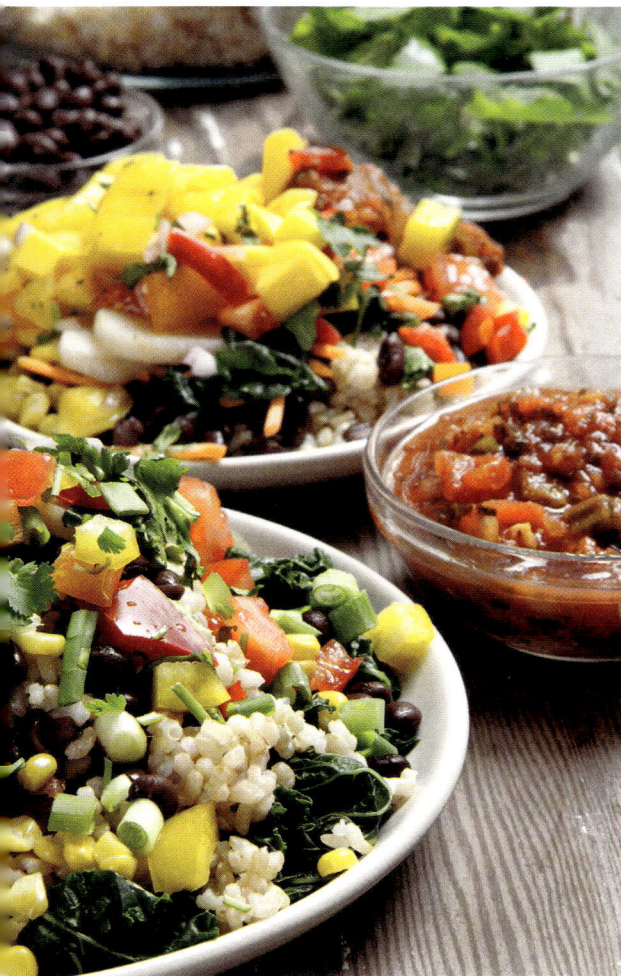

NOTE:

If you are lucky enough to have anything left over, stir it all together into a salad the next day with some salsa or some balsamic vinegar.

RICE, BEANS, AND GREENS
ON THE GO GO GO

This is easy and fast to prepare and turns out to be one of the dinners we eat most frequently. If you have leftover rice and just heat the beans under hot water, there is only the kale to cook! What could be quicker! And if you have an extra moment, add Corn Tortilla Taco Shells and Tostados (page 32) to the mix.

INGREDIENTS:

1 cup rice

2 cups water, or 1 cup vegetable broth and 1 cup water

1 (15-ounce) can no-salt-added black beans, drained and rinsed

1 cup cilantro, chopped

1 bunch kale, collards, or Swiss chard, stems stripped and leaves chopped into
   bite-size pieces

1 tomato, cored and chopped

1 green onion, chopped

Salsa, your favorite, for serving

INSTRUCTIONS:

Put the rice and water in a rice cooker or pot and cook according to the package directions. Warm beans in a small saucepan. Add ½ cup water and the cilantro, and stir to combine.

Bring 2 inches of water to boil in a large saucepan and add the kale. Cover and cook for 2 to 4 minutes, depending on how well-cooked you like your kale. Drain and rinse. (Alternatively, add the greens to the rice after the rice has been cooking for 25 minutes and skip this step.)

Put the kale on a plate, top with rice, beans, tomato, green onions, and salsa. Make a big green salad, and dinner is perfect.

MATT'S SOFRITO BLACK BEANS

I will never forget when our good friend Matt first served this dish to us! I thought I knew my way around black beans until I dined on this creation. A whole meal is based on these flavor-filled, beautifully textured beans. The key is using dry black beans and making the sofrito *(a mixture of yummy aromatic ingredients cut into small pieces and cooked together). Matt clearly told me, "No, Jane, you cannot use canned black beans. They'll disintegrate into a nasty mess." Aside from the time involved in prepping the beans, I cannot believe how easy this dish is and how well it turns out! Matt originally adapted this from* The Best Recipe. *He says emphatically that the salt in this dish is not optional (we did reduce it by half, though!). We often add Corn Tortilla Taco Shells and Tostados (page 32) to the table as my husband loves the added crunch with every bite.*

FOR THE BEANS:

- 1 pound dried black beans
- 1 green bell pepper, seeded and diced
- 1 medium onion, minced
- 6 cloves garlic, minced
- 2 bay leaves
- 1 teaspoon salt

FOR THE SOFRITO:

- 1 medium onion, minced
- 1 green bell pepper, seeded and minced
- 8 cloves garlic, minced
- 2 teaspoons dried oregano
- ½ teaspoon salt
- 1½ teaspoon ground cumin
- 1 tablespoon fresh lime juice
- 6 cups cooked brown rice, for serving

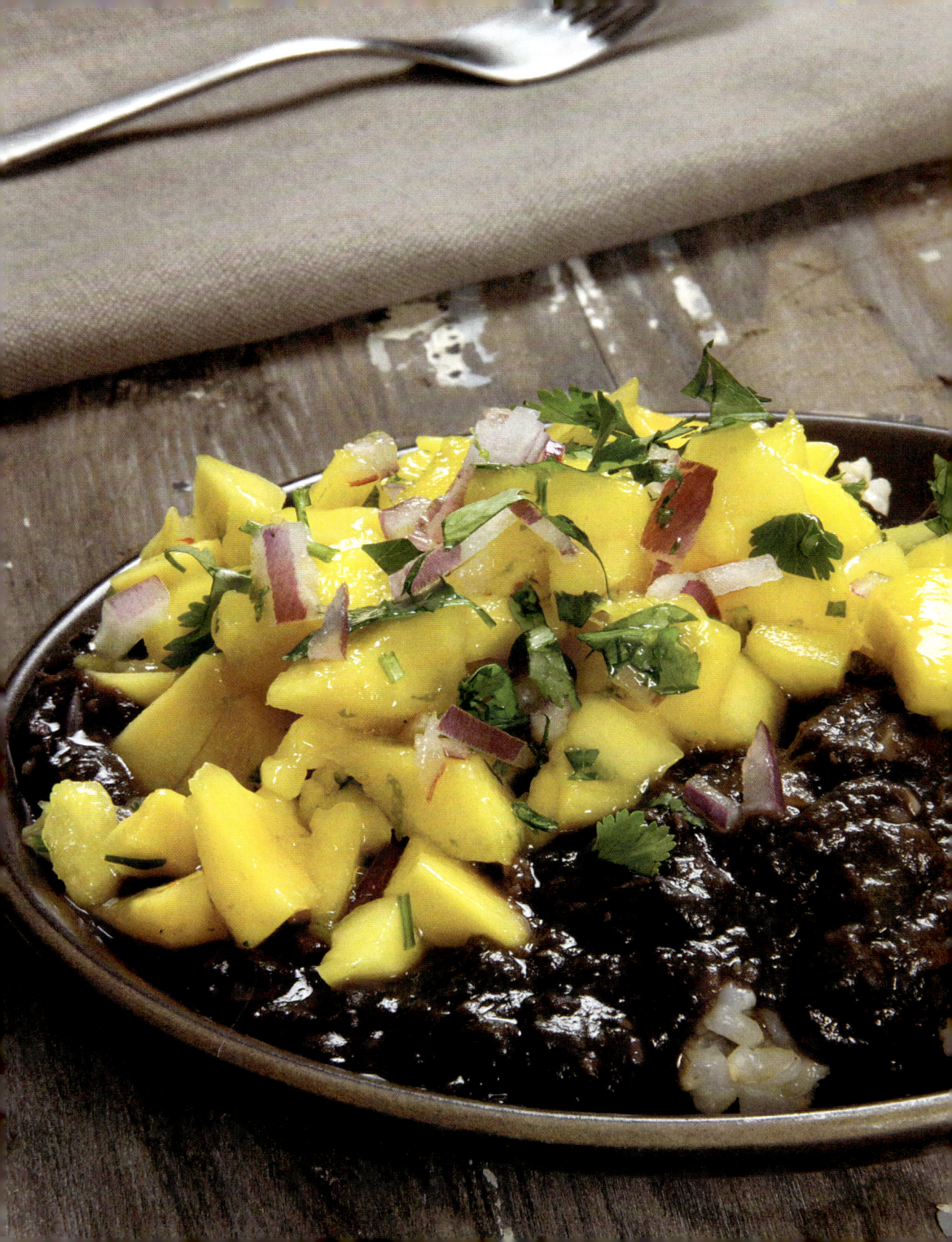

In a large soup pot, combine all the bean ingredients with 11 cups of water and bring the water to a boil over medium-high heat. Reduce the heat to low and simmer uncovered for 2 hours. At this point, the beans will be tender but not splitting. At the end of the 2-hour cooking time, remove and discard the bay leaves.

Close to the end of the beans' cooking time, start the sofrito. In a frying pan, cook the onions, bell pepper, garlic, oregano, and salt over medium-high heat, stirring. After 2 to 3 minutes, reduce the heat to medium. Continue to cook, stirring, as the vegetables soften, 8 to 10 minutes. Add a teaspoon of water whenever the pan gets too dry, and it will lift off the stuck-on sofrito. Add the cumin and stir until fragrant, about 1 minute more.

Add the sofrito to the beans. Using an immersion blender, fork, or potato masher, blend the mixture until about one-third to one-half of the beans are mashed—be wary of overblending. Blend a little, then stop and test. You want to preserve some of the whole beans yet create a mixture that is sort of uniformly smooth.

Simmer the beans over medium heat until the liquid has reduced and thickened, about 6 minutes. The beans will be creamy and the liquid will thicken to a saucelike consistency. Add the lime juice and simmer for 1 minute more.

Serve these flavorful beans over brown rice or alongside a big green salad. Our favorite way to serve this is over brown rice with Mango-Lime Salsa (page 120).

This dish gets thicker the next day, so we like to eat it with brown rice on the first day and in burritos or in the Matthew Wrap (page 74) the next day.

BLACK BEAN AND SWEET POTATO–COLLARD BURRITO

This recipe works equally well with collards or with whole-grain or brown rice wraps.

INGREDIENTS:

2 medium sweet potatoes, peeled, if desired, and chopped (6 to 8 cups)

1 onion, chopped

2 (15-ounce) cans no-salt-added black beans, drained and rinsed

½ cup vegetable broth

2 cloves garlic, chopped

1½ tablespoons chili powder

2 teaspoons Dijon mustard or mustard of choice

1 teaspoon ground cumin

⅛ teaspoon freshly ground black pepper

2 to 3 cups pasta sauce

6 medium collard leaves, stems trimmed

1 cup salsa, plus more as needed

1 cup chopped fresh cilantro or parsley

1 cup diced green onions

Fresh spinach, for serving

3 tablespoons nutritional yeast

INSTRUCTIONS:

Preheat the oven to 450°F.

Bring a large pot of water to a boil and cook the sweet potatoes until soft, about 10 minutes. Alternatively, bake them in the oven until cooked through, if preferred.

In a saucepan, cook the onions over medium heat for about 5 minutes, or until translucent. If the pan gets dry, add a few drops of water.

Add black beans, vegetable broth, garlic, chili powder, mustard, cumin, and pepper, and bring the mixture to a boil. Reduce the heat to medium and cook for 15 minutes.

Drain the water from sweet potatoes, mash them, and set aside.

In a baking dish or lasagna pan, spread 2 cups of the pasta sauce over the bottom of the dish; use more sauce if needed to cover the bottom of the dish.

In a large frying pan, bring 2 inches of water to a boil. Dunk the collard leaves one at a time in the boiling water for about 30 seconds, until flexible. Spread out the collards on the counter and pat both sides dry.

In the center of each collard leaf, place a line of mashed sweet potato (about ⅓ cup) topped with a line of black beans (about ⅓ cup), then 2 tablespoons salsa, a sprinkle of cilantro and green onions, and finally a small handful of spinach.

Fold over the tip of the leaf, then fold over the stem end of the leaf, and then fold in one side. Finally, roll the collard over the last side to create a burrito shape and place each little green collard burrito in the sauce-lined baking dish.

Cover with salsa or more pasta sauce and sprinkle the top with nutritional yeast.

Bake in the oven for 10 minutes or until warmed through.

SHRAPNEL BURRITO

General Henry Shrapnel invented the exploding hollow cannonball filled with shot and metal fragments. He named his invention "spherical case ammunition," yet we all know it as shrapnel. This recipe wraps up the plant-based fragments and scraps of almost anything in the shell of a burrito. Trust that when you combine the bits and pieces—the shrapnel—of what is in your fridge, it will all come together in a medley that tastes great. Here is what we often load our cannon with around here.

INGREDIENTS:

1½ cups cooked brown rice

4 ounces cherry tomatoes, halved

1 small zucchini, sliced

1 beet, peeled, cooked, and cubed

½ cup shredded carrot

1 (4-ounce) can green chiles, diced

1 (15-ounce) can no-salt-added black beans, drained and rinsed

1 (15-ounce) can no-fat vegetarian refried beans

Vegetables of your choice, diced

4 to 6 whole wheat, brown rice, or sprouted-grain wraps

INSTRUCTIONS:

Preheat the oven to 350°F.

In a large nonstick pan, stir together the rice, tomatoes, zucchini, beets, carrots, green chiles, black beans, and refried beans over medium-high heat. Add any other vegetables you want to add.

Scoop up the ingredients and place in the center of a wrap. Fold up the sides and wrap the burrito in foil. Repeat with the remaining wraps and filling.

Bake the burritos for 15 minutes.

Serve warm with your favorite salsas. We recommend Pico de Gallo (page 119), Mango-Lime Salsa (page 120), and Pomegranate Salsa (page 124).

SINGAPORE DAL

We first had this dal in Singapore. I stood right beside the chef so I wouldn't miss any of her secrets. The colors and the spices and the smells are embedded in my head. Putting the chiles in whole gives just the right amount of heat. This is delicious and thick over brown rice or potatoes. Serve it with a huge green salad or add Corn Tortilla Taco Shells and Tostados (page 32) instead of rice—or along with the rice! Fresh mango adds that last just-right touch.

INGREDIENTS:

- 1 onion, chopped
- 3 cloves garlic, chopped
- 2 tablespoons chopped, peeled fresh ginger
- 1 teaspoon ground coriander
- 1 teaspoon ground cumin
- 1 teaspoon garam masala
- 3 medium tomatoes, cored and chopped
- 1 (15-ounce) can no-salt-added black-eyed peas, drained and rinsed
- 1 (15-ounce) can no-salt-added chickpeas or any white bean, drained and rinsed
- 2 cups vegetable stock or water
- 3 small skinny green chiles (also called finger chiles; serrano chiles will work, too)
- 1 tablespoon fresh lemon juice
- Chopped fresh cilantro, for serving
- 1 mango, chopped, for serving

INSTRUCTIONS:

In a saucepan, cook the onions over medium heat until they begin to soften; then add the garlic and ginger and continue to cook, stirring, for a few more minutes. Add drops of water as necessary if the pan gets dry. Add the coriander, cumin, and garam masala, and cook for 2 minutes more for flavors to mingle. Again, add a few drops of water if the pan gets dry. Add the tomatoes, black-eyed peas, chickpeas, vegetable stock, and whole green chiles! Bring the mixture to a boil, reduce the heat to maintain a simmer, and cook until the dal has thickened to a gravylike consistency, about 30 minutes. Add the lemon juice and lots of cilantro. Before serving, remove the chiles, or if you want more heat, break up the chiles and add them to the dish to suit your taste. Serve with chopped fresh mango in every bite. Perfection!

NORI NOIR–BLACK RICE–FILLED NORI ROLLS

MAKES 4 NORI ROLLS (25 TO 30 PIECES)

My mom called me from a loud, crowded event to tell me about these spectacular nori rolls! She was over the moon about the "cat's-eyes contrast of the yellow pepper and the black rice." Now we make these high-contrast rolls when we want to show off! These are equally delicious using short-grain brown rice, just not quite as cat's-eye stunning.

INGREDIENTS:

2 cups cooked black rice (this tends to be sticky, which is good for this recipe!)

2 tablespoons brown rice vinegar (optional)

1 package nori sheets (usually contains 7 to 10 sheets)

1 yellow bell pepper, seeded and julienned

2 green onions, chopped

½ cucumber, peeled, seeded, and cut lengthwise into thin strips

2 long carrots, shredded

8 spears asparagus, steamed

1 mango, pitted, peeled, and cut into strips

Wasabi powder

Pickled ginger

Low-sodium tamari

INSTRUCTIONS:

Place the cooked black rice in a large bowl and stir. If the rice is not sticky, stir in the brown rice vinegar until the texture becomes sticky.

Place 1 sheet of nori flat on a dry surface. Spread about ½ cup of the black rice on one-half of the flat sheet (like covering half of a tennis court).

Place the vegetables of your choice and mango horizontally in the middle of the flattened rice. Using both hands, starting from the rice-covered end, roll up the sheet. Carefully cover the vegetables and keep rolling. The roll will stick to itself especially well if the rice is still a little warm. If your nori does not stick, try dabbing the edge of the non-rice-covered end with water.

Slice each roll crosswise with a sharp knife into ½-inch medallion-style pieces.

Make the desired amount of wasabi paste by adding water to the wasabi powder as directed on the package.

Serve the nori pieces with little dishes of pickled ginger, wasabi paste, and tamari. Dip each nori roll in one or all of the little dishes. Or eat them just as they are.

VARIATION:

Use other colored whole-grain rice instead of black rice.

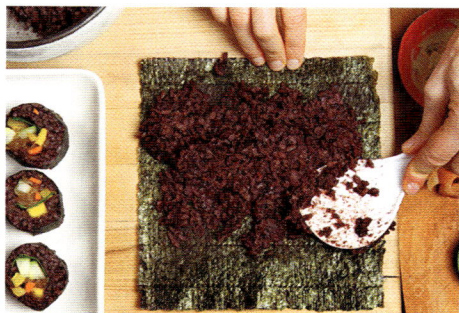

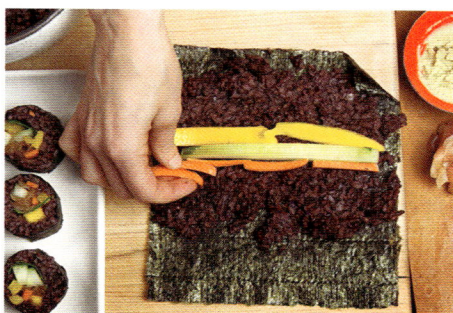

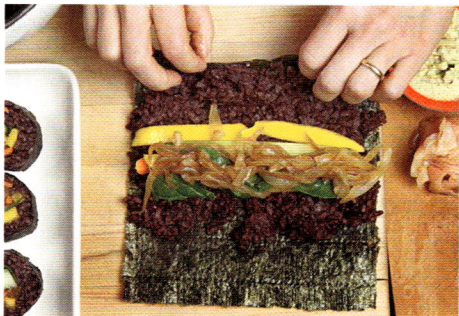

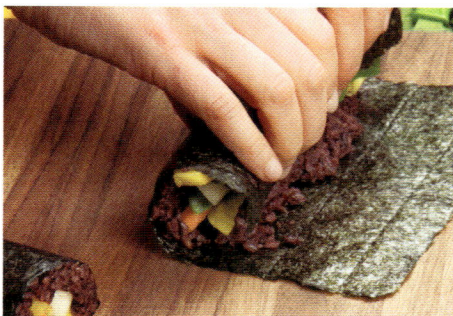

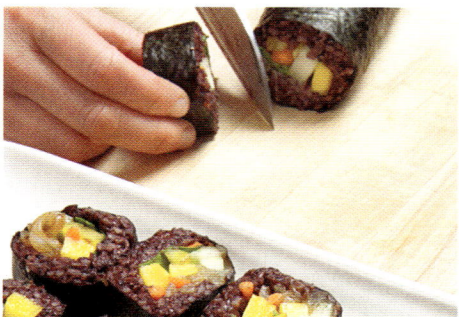

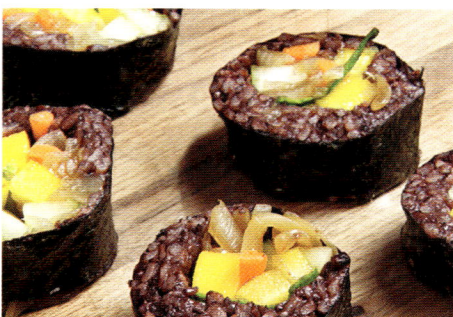

CHILE RELLENOS

During her brief visit, our friend Norma showed us how to make these and many other traditional Mexican dishes. It felt as if we were learning magic tricks! Chile rellenos was a dish we had only experienced in restaurants! And voilà—here we suddenly were making them ourselves—at home! Serve these stunning beauties with quinoa or brown rice and a huge salad.

INGREDIENTS:

6 poblano peppers

16 ounces no-fat vegetarian refried beans or mashed pinto beans

2 tomatoes (or 1 large tomato), quartered

¼ onion, chopped

3 cups Enchilada Sauce (page 114), Mango-Lime Salsa (page 120), Roasted Tomatillo Salsa (page 122), or Pico de Gallo (page 119)

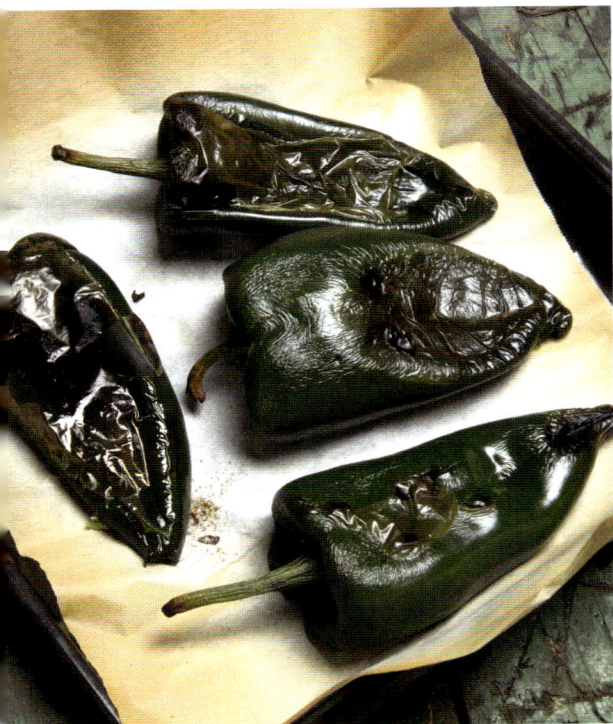

INSTRUCTIONS:

Roast the peppers over the stovetop, or on a pan in the oven on broil. Rotate the peppers until the skin burns and evenly releases from the pepper flesh. Place peppers in a plastic bag, seal, and wrap in a towel for at least 10 minutes. This helps the skin to release.

Remove the peppers from the bag and peel off the skin. Cut a line an inch or two from the crown of the pepper toward the tip. Open the incision and remove the seeds and white veins inside.

Into each pepper, spoon 2 to 3 tablespoons of refried beans. Press the pepper flesh closed, and place the stuffed peppers aside on a platter.

Place the tomatoes, onions, and 1 cup water in a food processor, and blend for 2 to 3 minutes, until the sauce is light pink and quite liquidy. This we will call chile rellenos sauce.

Fill a medium saucepan with the chile rellenos

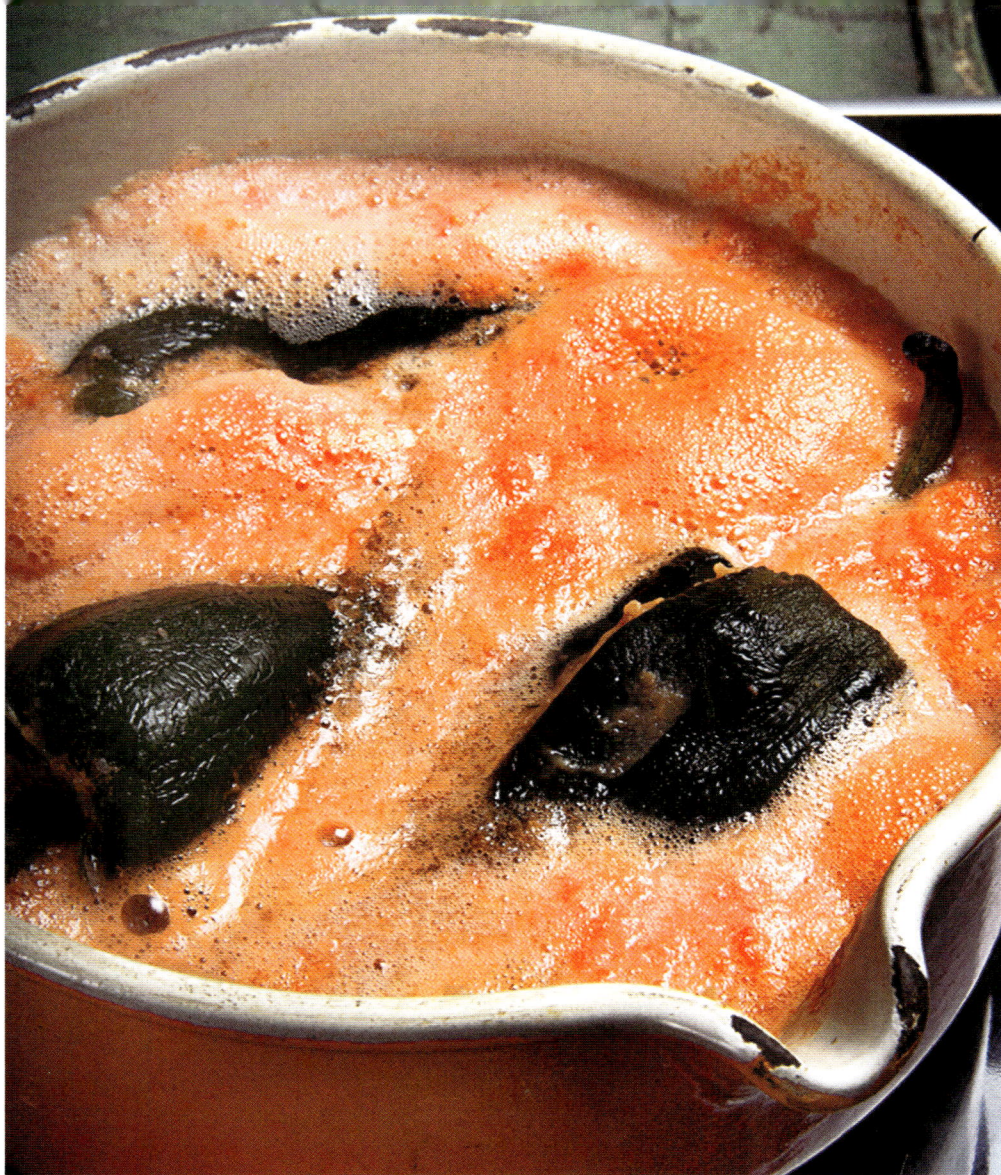

sauce and set it over medium heat. Place the stuffed peppers into the pan and simmer for 15 minutes.

Remove the peppers from the saucepan and serve immediately over quinoa or brown rice, with the sauces or salsas of your choice!

The extra chile rellenos sauce can be used however you wish—be inventive.

STUFFED PORTOBELLO CAPS

These beautiful stuffed portobello mushrooms alone are a lovely center of the main course, or serve them on top of brown rice along with a large salad. They are beautiful when they are draped with Roasted Red Peppers (page 24). If you don't make your own peppers, no-oil jarred roasted peppers are available but do not have the same delicious, marinated flavor as ours. We urge you to make your own—you will become as addicted as we are!

INGREDIENTS:

- 2 portobello mushrooms
- 2 tablespoons balsamic vinegar
- 3 to 4 cloves garlic, crushed
- ½ cup vegetable broth
- 1 bunch Swiss chard, leaves and stems chopped
- 4 tablespoons Our Hummus (page 102) or hummus prepared without oil or tahini
- 2 green onions, chopped (about ¼ cup)
- 1 teaspoon Dijon mustard
- 6 to 8 red pepper strips (see Roasted Red Peppers, page 24)

INSTRUCTIONS:

Preheat the oven to 400°F.

Remove the stems and gills from the portobello mushrooms (a spoon works well for this), reserving the stems and discarding the gills. Place the mushroom caps hollow-side up in a baking dish.

Roughly chop the portobello stems and put them in the baking dish alongside the mushroom caps.

Fill each portobello center with 1 tablespoon of the balsamic vinegar and half the garlic, and mix gently in the caps. Pour vegetable broth in the bottom of the baking dish.

Bake for 10 minutes. Remove the dish from the oven and set it aside; leave the oven on.

Bring 3 inches of water to a boil in a large pot and cook the Swiss chard for 3 minutes, or until soft. Drain.

In a bowl, combine the hummus, green onions, and Dijon mustard, and stir. Remove the cooked mushroom stems from the baking dish, chop them into small pieces, and mix them in with the hummus and green onions.

Fill each mushroom cap with a heaping ¼ cup of Swiss chard, and sprinkle the Swiss chard with a tablespoon of juice from the bottom of the portobello baking dish. Top this growing creation with some of the hummus mixture and 3 red pepper strips.

Return the baking dish to the oven and bake for 10 minutes more, until the hummus is bubbling. Before serving, sprinkle the stuffed mushrooms with green onions. Any extra juice in the bottom of the pan may be poured over the mushrooms for an extra little kiss of flavor.

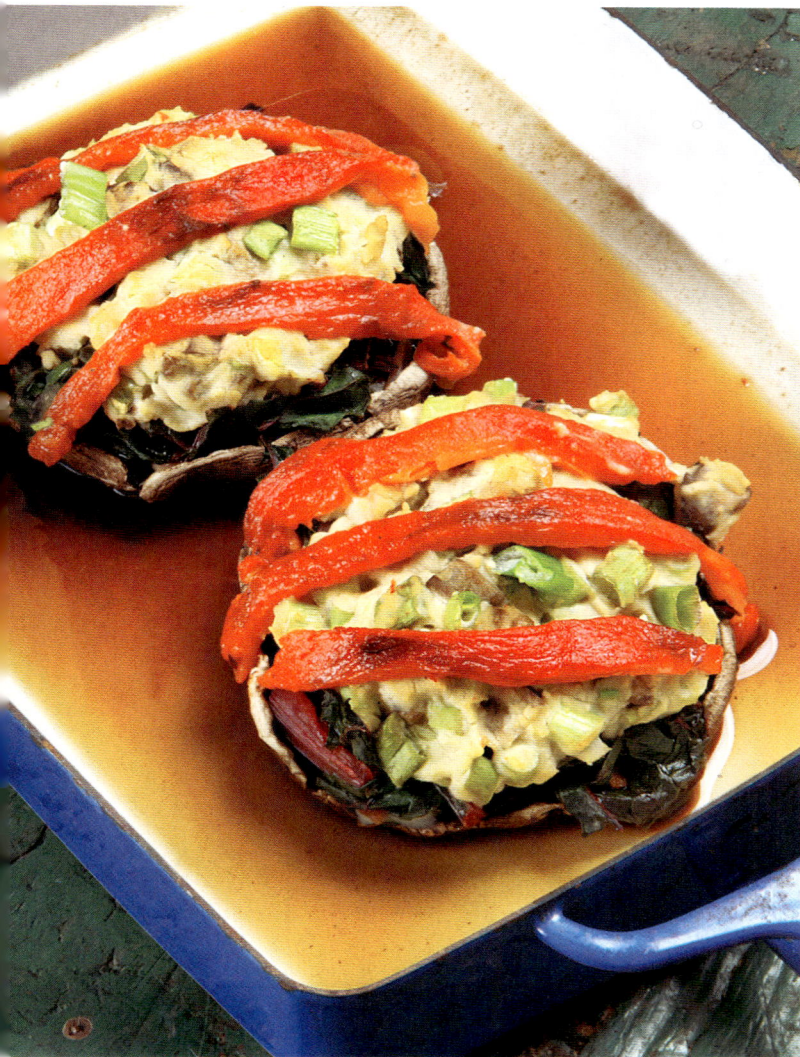

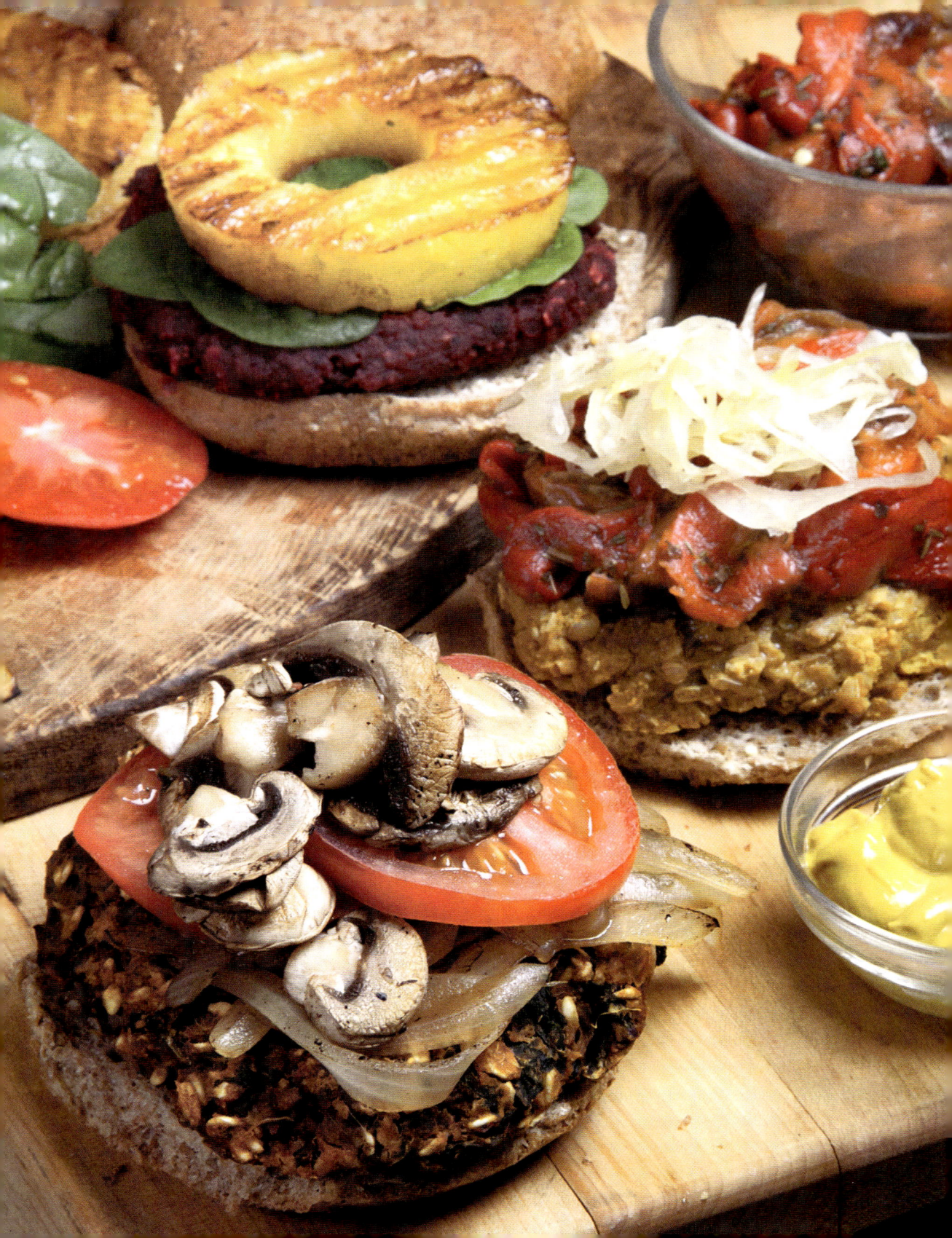

S.O.B. BURGERS–SMOKY, OAT, BEAN BURGERS

MAKES 6 BURGERS

My mom suggested using S.O.B. in the title. It makes me chuckle. Here is what she wrote: "Let's invent a burger and use liquid smoke or smoky paprika and have oats and beans in it. We could call them Smoky, Oat, Bean Burgers: S.O.B. Burgers! Ha!" Here they are.

INGREDIENTS:

½ cup short-grain brown rice

1 cup vegetable broth

½ cup nutritional yeast

2 (15-ounce) cans no-salt-added cannellini beans, drained and rinsed

¼ cup old-fashioned rolled oats

¼ cup salsa, as hot as you can handle

½ teaspoon turmeric

1 teaspoon onion powder

1 teaspoon garlic powder

½ teaspoon smoky paprika

¼ teaspoon liquid smoke (optional)

Six 100 percent whole-grain buns

Fixings: Mustard, ketchup, relish, tomato slices, red onion slices, spinach, romaine, sauerkraut, Roasted Red Peppers (page 24), Sautéed Mushrooms (page 28), Caramelized Onions (page 26)

INSTRUCTIONS:

Preheat the oven to 350°F if you choose to bake and not pan-fry the burgers. We make them both ways and don't have a preference. Sometimes it is the busy stovetop or occupied oven that dictates.

Line a sheet pan with parchment paper.

In a rice cooker or in a pot on the stovetop, combine the rice and vegetable broth, and cook as directed. When the rice is done, transfer it to a bowl and stir while the rice is still warm and moist. The rice will get stickier and stickier the more you stir.

Into the rice mixture add the nutritional yeast, cannellini beans, oats, and salsa. Using your hands smash, smash, smash until none of the skins of the beans are intact. *Really* smash and squeeze the beans.

Add the turmeric, onion powder, garlic powder, smoky paprika, and liquid smoke, and continue to hand-mix and mash. The mixture will be quite mortarlike.

Form the mixture into patties.

Place the patties in a nonstick frying pan over medium heat and cook for 5 minutes per side, or bake for 20 minutes, 10 minutes per side, until warmed through.

Serve with your choice of fixings!

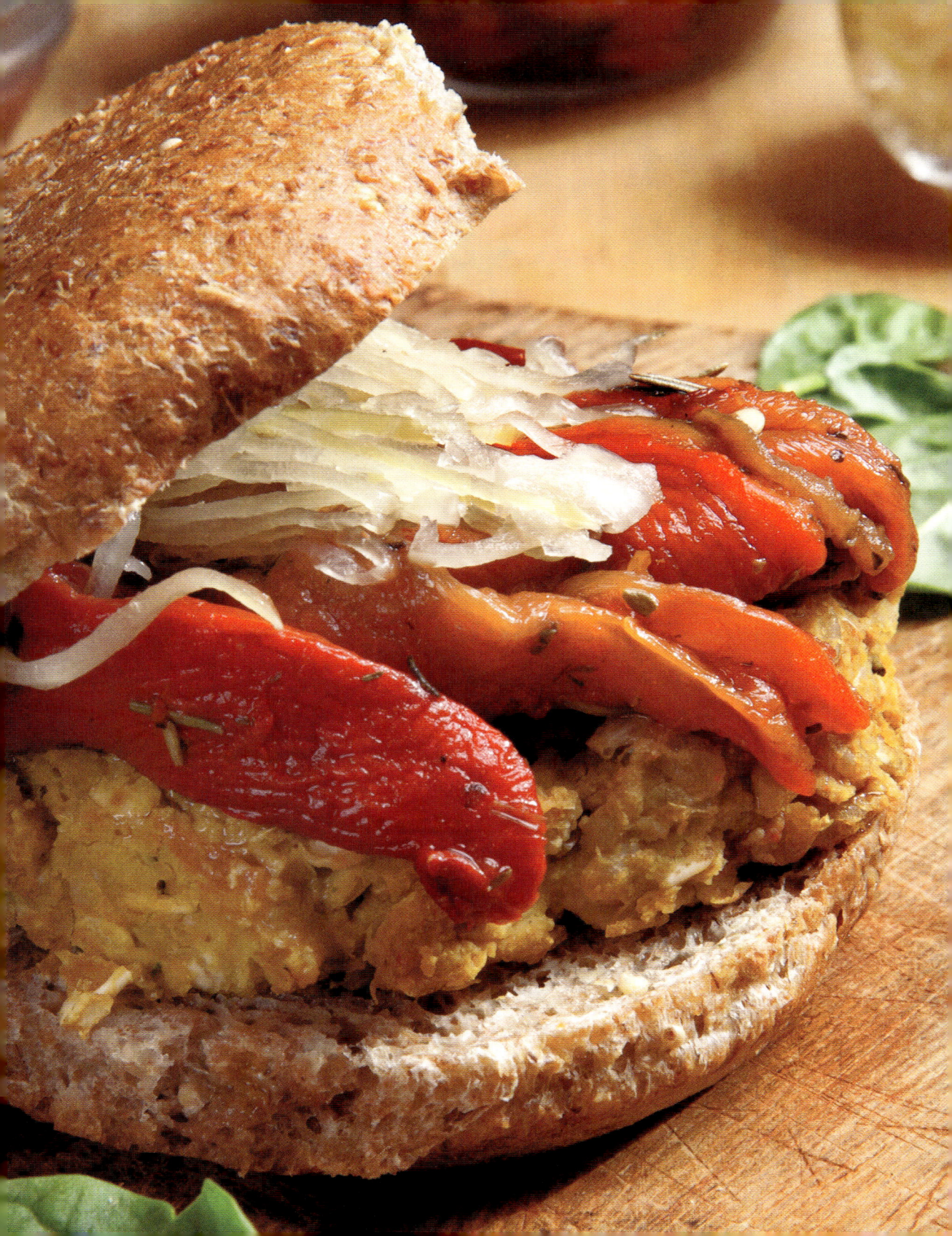

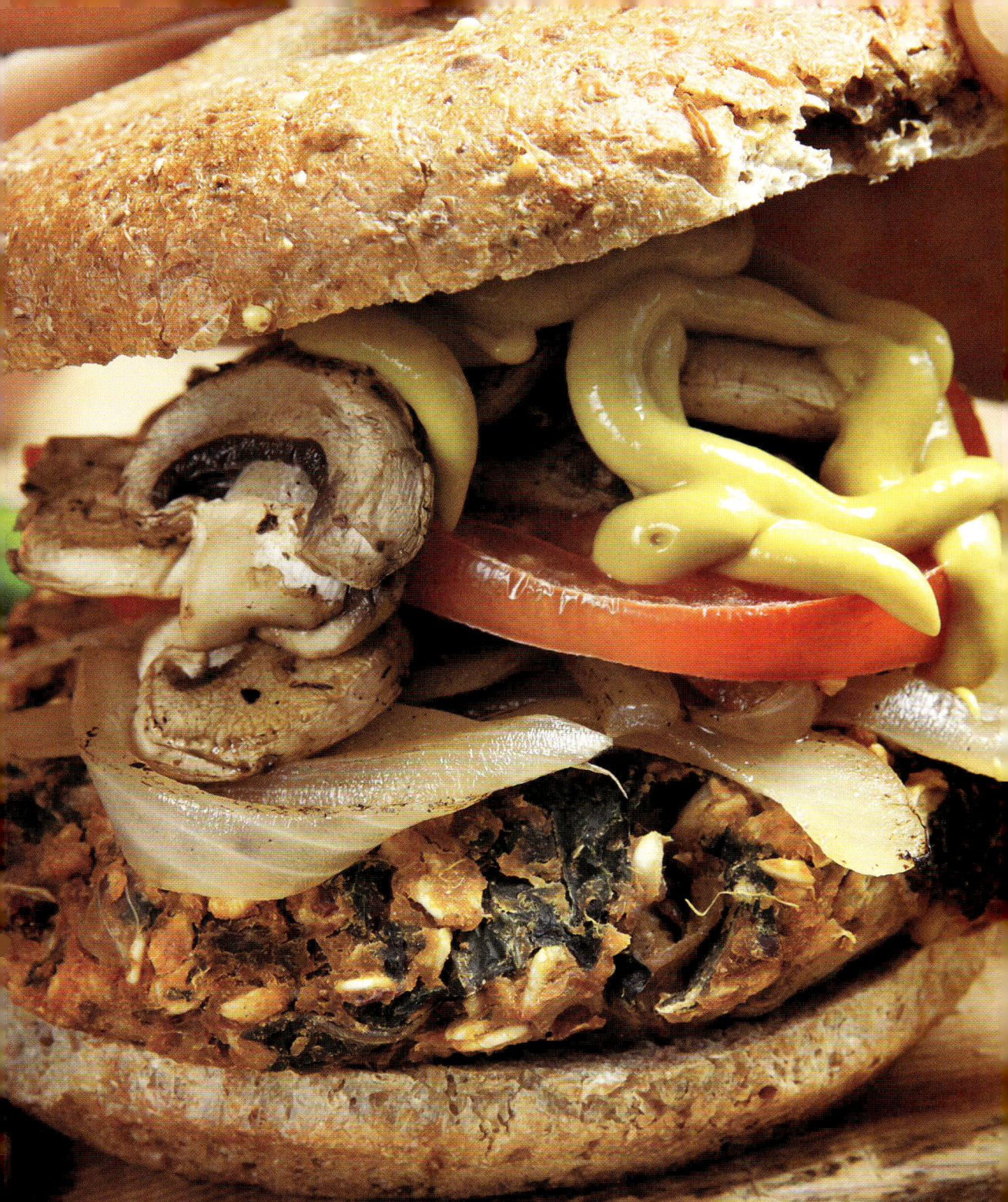

KALE BURGER

For many of us, a burger is just a vehicle for ketchup, mustard, and the other fixings. Yet these kale burgers bring great taste and texture to the equation as well! This recipe is one of our favorites because it sticks together and has kale in it.

INGREDIENTS:

1 cup diced onion

2 large cloves garlic, minced

8 ounces mushrooms, sliced (optional)

1 cup kale, free of spines and shredded into tiny pieces

1 medium sweet potato, cooked and removed from skin

1 cup old-fashioned oats

2 (15-ounce) cans no-salt-added kidney beans, drained and rinsed

2 tablespoons sriracha hot chili sauce, Tabasco sauce, or similar hot sauce

Six to eight 100 percent whole-grain buns

Fixings: Mustard, ketchup, relish, tomato slices, red onion slices, spinach, romaine, sauerkraut, Roasted Red Peppers (page 24), Sautéed Mushrooms (page 28), Caramelized Onions (page 26)

INSTRUCTIONS:

In a hot frying pan, so hot that a drop of water beads across the surface, cook the onions, and garlic, stirring consistently until browned slightly and cooked throughout. Reduce the heat to medium and add the mushrooms and kale and continue stirring.

After the mushrooms are cooked thoroughly and the kale turns dark green, turn off the heat and set aside.

In a large bowl, smash and mix together the sweet potato, oats, kidney beans, and sriracha sauce.

Add the cooked vegetables to the bowl and continue mixing—hands work best!

Using your hands, form the mixture into patties.

Place the patties on a nonstick frying pan over medium-low heat for 20 minutes, 10 minutes per side, or until browned on the outside and warmed through. Serve with your choice of fixings!

BEET BURGERS WITH GRILLED PINEAPPLE

Essy and I were treated to an amazing beet burger lunch created and prepared by three enthusiastic plant-based Ohio University students. We were blown away by the unique flavor of these burgers and by Gabe, Chance, and David for their incredible enthusiasm for plant-based eating. They helped us tweak their recipe just right; a delicious red, meaty-looking burger that holds together well. The most fun of all is the very red hands you get while making these! Just wait! (But no worries, the bright red washes right off.) With Grilled Pineapple (page 29), sauerkraut, or any of your favorite toppings, these burgers are truly stunners! Thank you, Gabe, Chance, and David!

INGREDIENTS:

3 large beets, including greens and stems

3 cloves garlic, roughly chopped

1 cup nutritional yeast

1 cup cooked brown rice or cooked quinoa

1 cup old-fashioned oats

1 tablespoon onion flakes

1 tablespoon garlic flakes

1½ teaspoons wasabi powder

1 (15-ounce) can no-salt-added kidney beans, drained and rinsed

Grilled Pineapple (page 29)

Eight to ten 100 percent whole wheat buns

Fixings: Mustard, ketchup, relish, tomato slices, red onion slices, spinach, romaine, sauerkraut

INSTRUCTIONS:

Preheat oven to 400° F. Line a sheet pan with parchment paper.

Remove both ends of the beets, rinse well, chop into ½-inch-thick slices, place them on the prepared sheet pan, and bake for 20 to 30 minutes or until tender.

Rinse the beet greens and roughly chop the stems and greens. In a pot with a few inches of water, boil the beet greens and stems for about 3 minutes, until tender. Drain and set aside. If the beets don't have good greens, some Swiss chard will work.

Put the beets and garlic in the food processor and blend briefly until roughly chopped and in tiny chunks. Don't over-blend.

Add the nutritional yeast and well-drained beet greens and pulse until barely incorporated. Don't over-pulse or the batter will turn to hummus. (It will still work, but it won't make as nice a burger.)

In a large bowl, combine brown rice, oats, onion flakes, garlic flakes, and wasabi powder, and stir to mix in evenly.

Add the kidney beans. With your hands, massage the beans into the rice and oats, until roughly combined.

Now the real fun begins! Add the beet mixture and continue to mix it all together with your hands. Keep the texture of the mixture sort of rough. You will have very red hands!

Make a small snowball with the batter.

In a nonstick pan over medium-low heat, place the red ball and press down with your hand from the center. The batter should spread out evenly and come to fruition as a beautiful-looking beet patty. Cook for about 5 minutes on each side, on nothing higher than medium to medium-low heat. These unique burgers taste best when they are cooked through, which can only be accomplished on lower heats. Nothing can beat these in a whole wheat bun topped with Grilled Pineapple and sauerkraut. They are also good plain with ketchup.

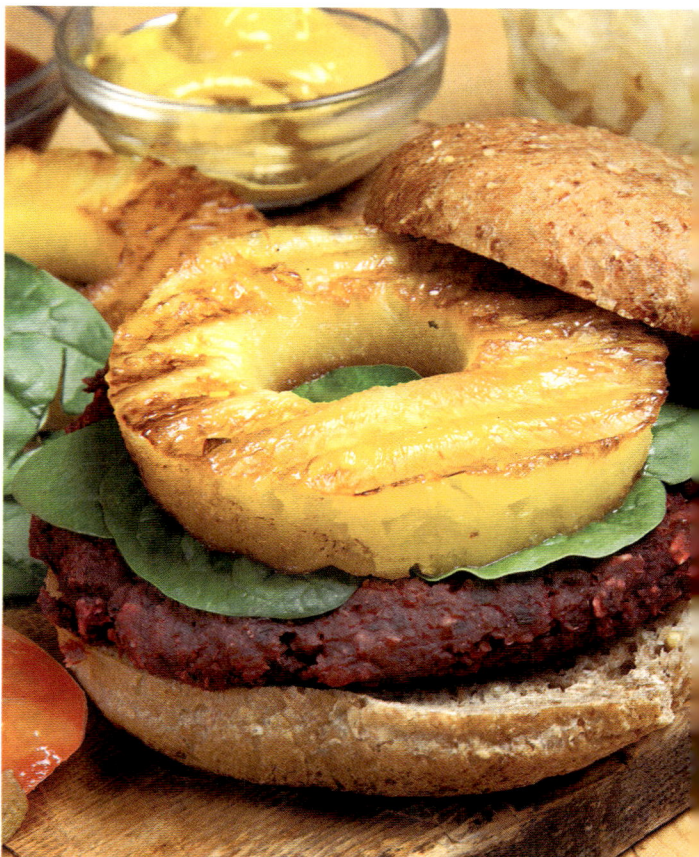

SLOPPY JOES AND TIDY JANES

What a comfort food—and so quick to make, especially if you have lentils ready to go. We enjoy Sloppy Joes on buns—you should see how fast my dad can gobble these up. Or sometimes we prefer the tidier version of these, which we call Tidy Janes. We serve the Tidy Jane version in Crispy Tortilla Bowls (page 30)—the flavor-soaked bowl is delicious if you eat it right afterward. Or try serving this yummy filling in Corn Tortilla Taco Shells and Tostados (page 32). However you serve these, eat them with a big green salad.

INGREDIENTS:

- 3 cups cooked brown lentils (or 1½ cups dry lentils and 3½ cups water)
- 1 medium onion, diced
- 1 red bell pepper, diced
- 1 cup mushrooms, sliced
- 6 ounces tomato paste
- 1 (15-ounce) can diced tomatoes (drained)
- 4 tablespoons barbecue sauce (we prefer Bone Suckin' Sauce)
- ¼ teaspoon liquid smoke (optional)
- 1 teaspoon pure maple syrup
- 2 teaspoons chili powder
- 4 whole wheat buns, if making Sloppy Joes, or 4 whole wheat or brown rice tortillas, if making Tidy Janes or 8 to 10 Corn Tortilla Taco Shells and Tostados (page 32)

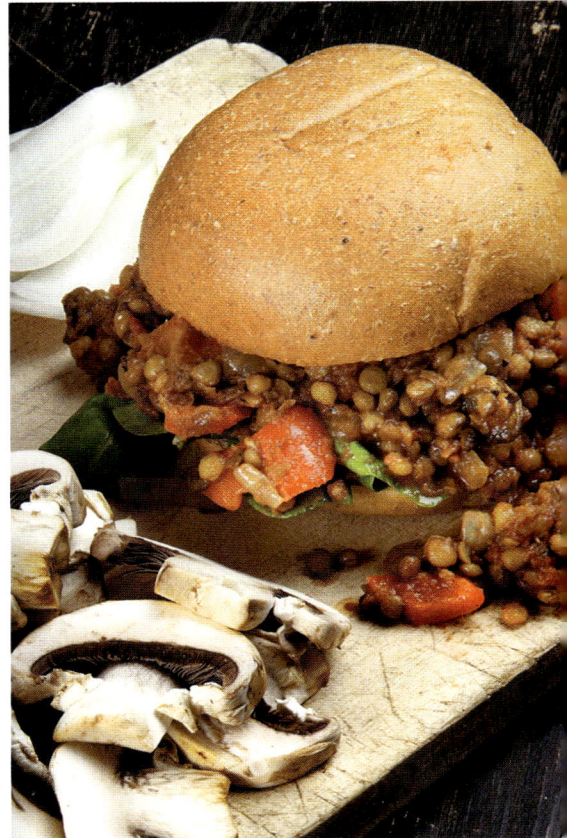

If you are starting with dry lentils, combine dry lentils and water in a pot. Bring to a boil; then simmer for 20 minutes until the lentils are soft. Drain if necessary.

In a frying pan over medium heat, cook the onions, pepper, and mushrooms until soft and slightly browned. Add the tomato paste and diced tomatoes and continue to stir over low heat. Add the cooked lentils, barbecue sauce, liquid smoke, maple syrup, and chili powder, and thoroughly mix. Reduce the heat to simmer for 5 more minutes.

Taste and tweak mixture to your liking: Add more maple syrup or barbecue sauce for a sweeter, smokier or more fiery flavor.

Generously spoon the mixture onto buns or into Crispy Tortilla Bowls!

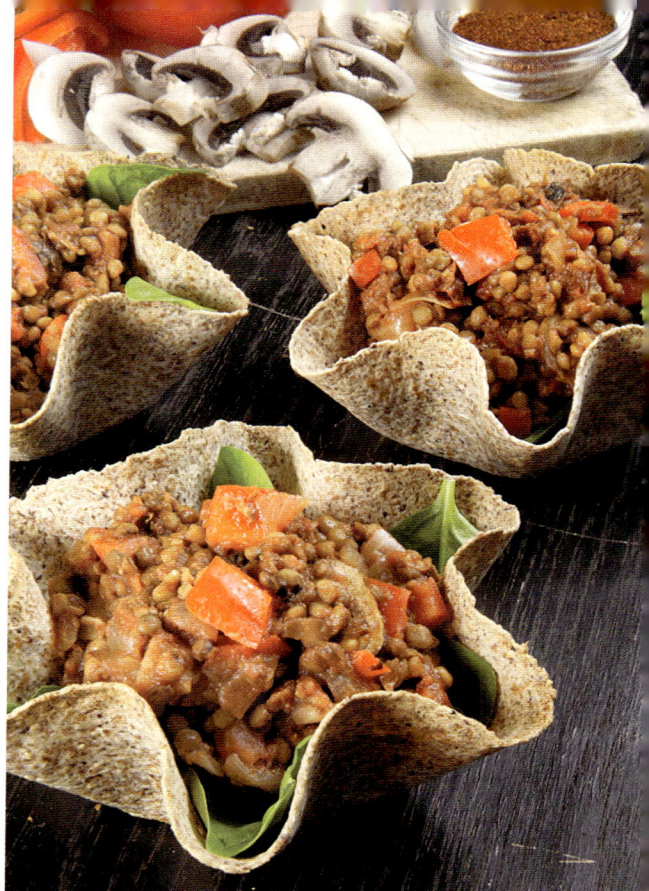

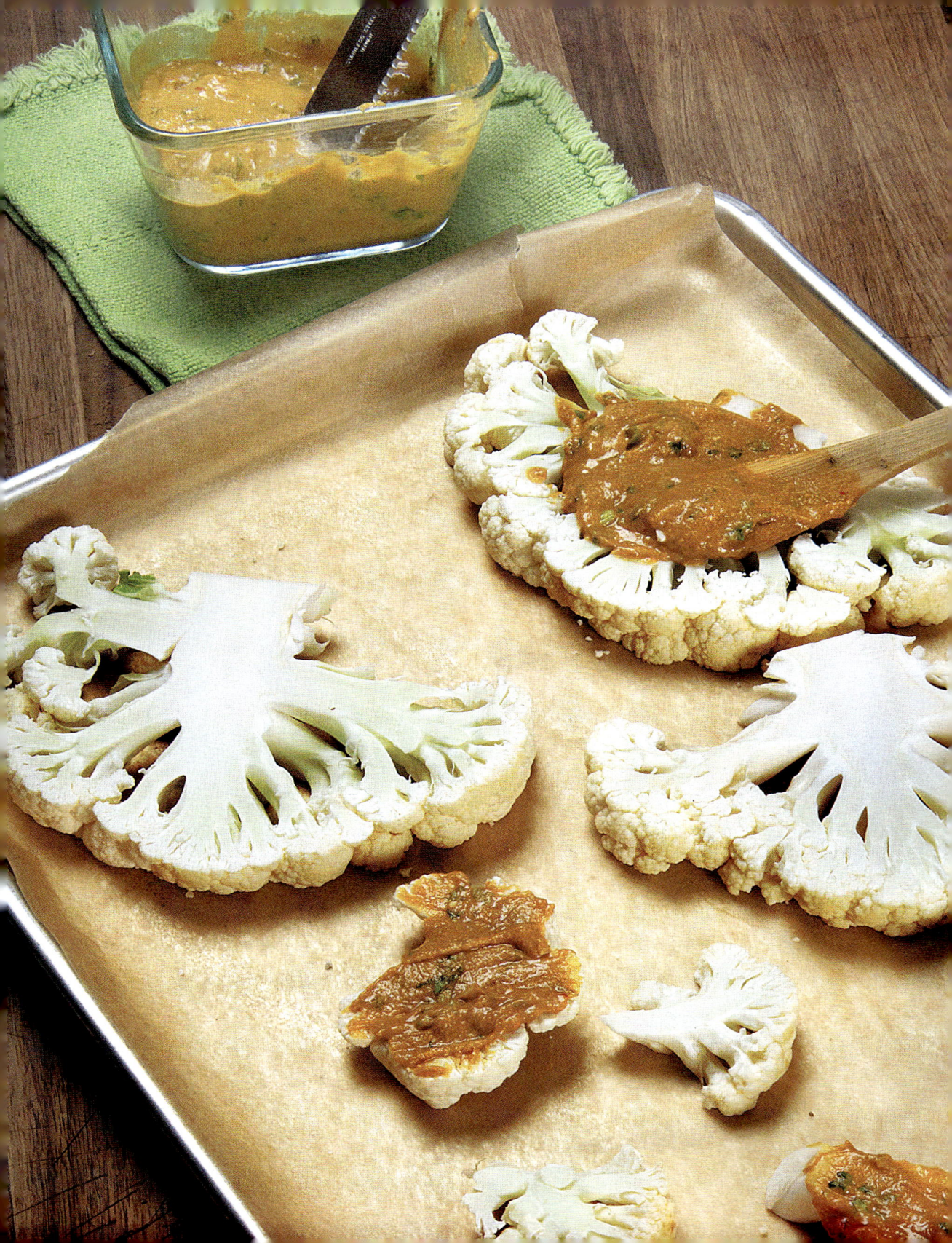

CAULIFLOWER STEAKS

These are amazing! *It's hard to say how many people this recipe serves since one person could easily eat them all. If you have a really large cauliflower and run out of sauce, leave some without since it is also good roasted plain. With a really large cauliflower, you may need two baking sheets. By the way, this sauce is a much better color using* white *balsamic vinegar. The sauce is delicious on its own or on anything you choose.*

INGREDIENTS:

- 1 head cauliflower (find a large one!)
- ½ cup Our Hummus (page 102) or hummus with no added oil or tahini
- ½ cup nutritional yeast
- 3 tablespoons balsamic vinegar, divided (white balsamic recommended)
- 2 tablespoons water
- 2 tablespoons green onions, chopped
- 2 tablespoons cilantro or parsley, chopped

INSTRUCTIONS:

Preheat oven to 450°F.

Line a sheet pan with parchment paper.

Cut a head of cauliflower in half, then cut about ½- to ¾-inch "steaks," about 4 to 6 in all, and place them flat on the prepared pan. Lots of tiny bits may fall apart; that is okay. Place them all on the pan.

Make the sauce. Combine the hummus, nutritional yeast, 2 tablespoons of balsamic vinegar, water, green onions, and cilantro, and stir. Spread this sauce over the cauliflower steaks and over the extra broken-up pieces. Sprinkle the remaining 1 tablespoon balsamic vinegar in thin lines over the top of all the coated cauliflower.

Bake for 30 minutes; check and continue baking longer if the steaks are not soft enough. The steaks should be soft and browned on top and bottom. Actually, the longer these cook, the better!

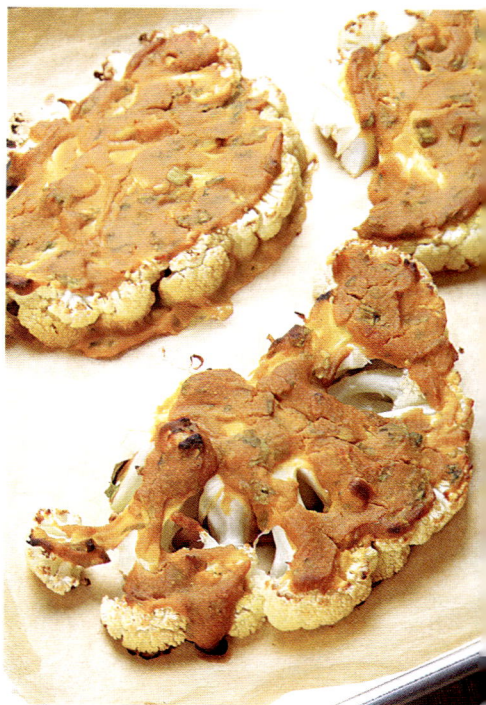

CAULIFLOWER BUFFALO "WINGS"

Two pals from different coasts told me about this new way of making wings, so we had to try it. Buffalo wings are spicy hot and usually served as an appetizer. But if you can take the heat, this whole dish is easy to eat as a meal! Make sure to have your salad and greens, too.

INGREDIENTS:

- 1 head cauliflower
- 1 cup chickpea flour
- 2 teaspoons garlic powder
- 1 teaspoon onion powder
- ¼ teaspoon black pepper
- 1 cup oat milk or almond milk
- 1½ cups hot sauce (we prefer Cholulu)

INSTRUCTIONS:

Preheat the oven to 400°F.

Line a sheet pan with parchment paper.

Cut a head of cauliflower into bite-size chunks.

In a bowl, mix together the chickpea flour, garlic powder, onion powder, black pepper, and oat milk. Stir the batter so there are no lumps.

Immerse the cauliflower pieces into the batter so they are well coated, and then place them on the lined pan. Cook for 18 minutes.

Take the pan out of the oven and drown (seriously) the cauliflower "wings" in your favorite hot sauce. Cook for another 8 minutes.

Dip these hot "wings" in your choice of dressings.

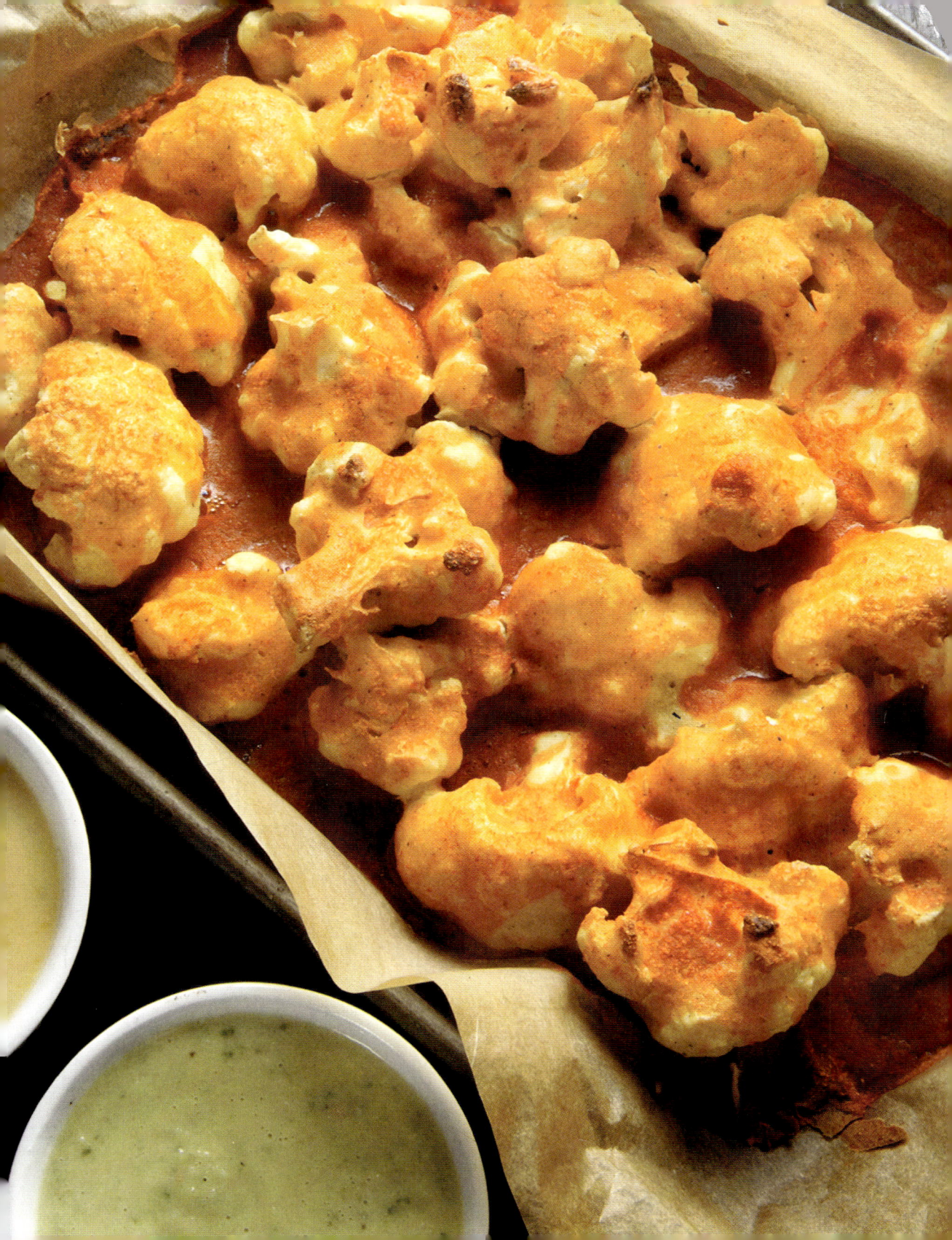

BBQ PORTOBELLOS, RICE, AND GREENS

I watched Jane prepare this in the morning so she could just pop it in the oven at the last minute for dinner. I went right home and made the same dinner for us. It is delicious with toasted corn tortillas and a green salad. We like Bone Suckin' Sauce, but use what you like. Avoid high-fructose corn syrup and make sure the brand you choose has tomatoes as the first ingredient. If you want to avoid the sugar, make your own sauce with tomato sauce and balsamic vinegar.

INGREDIENTS:

- 1 very large onion, sliced
- 2 tablespoons balsamic vinegar, vegetable broth, or water (to keep the pan moist)
- 4 portobello mushrooms
- ½ to 1 cup barbecue sauce of your choice
- 4 to 6 cups kale or other greens, stems removed and torn into bite-size pieces
- 4 cups cooked brown rice, warmed

INSTRUCTIONS:

Preheat the oven to 400°F.

Place the onions in the bottom of an 8 × 8-inch pan or any small casserole dish and add a few tablespoons of balsamic vinegar to the bottom of the pan. Arrange the portobello mushrooms gill-side up on top of the onions. Spread about 1 tablespoon barbecue sauce (or a bit more if you like) over the mushrooms, and bake for 40 minutes until the onions are nicely browned.

Place the kale in 2 to 3 inches of boiling water in a frying pan or pot, cover, and cook 4 to 6 minutes or until tender to your preference. Drain well.

In each bowl, place a layer of kale, warm rice, and a mushroom, and pile onions on top. Sprinkle with any extra juice from the pan. It is helpful to use a knife to cut the mushrooms.

MELLOW GINGER SAUCE OVER
CHICKPEAS AND GREENS

SERVES 6 TO 8

This dish is grounding and mellow. We love it, and believe it or not, it gets even better the next day. It makes a secret leftover to hide in the refrigerator so only you know it is there. If you choose to make this more like a soup, simply add more vegetable broth. Our daughter-in-law Polly calls this a healing stew!

INGREDIENTS:

3 large sweet onions, halved and thinly sliced

3 to 4 tablespoons ginger, chopped

3 (15-ounce) cans no-salt-added chickpeas

½ cup vegetable broth

⅛ teaspoon cayenne pepper or more to taste

4 to 5 tablespoons lemon juice plus zest of 1 lemon

2 cups or more fresh spinach

½ to 1 cup cilantro, chopped

INSTRUCTIONS:

In a large pan over medium-high heat, cook the onions about 15 minutes until soft and just beginning to brown.

Add the ginger and continue to stir for a few minutes more. Add a few drops of vegetable broth or water if the pan looks dry.

Add the chickpeas and the liquid from the can, along with the cayenne, and cover and simmer 25 minutes.

With a potato masher, fork, or spoon, mash some of the chickpeas right in the pan to create a thicker sauce.

Stir in the lemon juice and lemon zest, spinach, and cilantro. Serve over rice or quinoa on a bed of steamed greens and you have a lovely meal in one bowl. You can also eat the chickpeas just plain.

FAST PASTA AND GREENS

Use any whole-grain pasta, oil-free pasta sauce, greens, or vegetables you desire. Just be sure to fill that pasta pot, when the timer goes off, with lots of greens. This is such a good one-bowl meal and though it takes a number of pots, it is ready very quickly. Skip the zucchini and mushrooms if you are in a hurry. Then it is fast!

INGREDIENTS:

8 ounces whole wheat pasta

1 large bunch kale, collards, Swiss chard, or spinach (or a combination), stems removed, leaves chopped into bite-size pieces (6 to 8 cups)

16 ounces pasta sauce

1 zucchini, sliced

12 ounces mushrooms, sliced

INSTRUCTIONS:

In a pot of boiling water, cook the pasta for 3 minutes less than the directions recommend. Set a timer.

When the timer goes off, add the chopped kale to the pasta water so it will cook along with the pasta for the last 3 minutes.

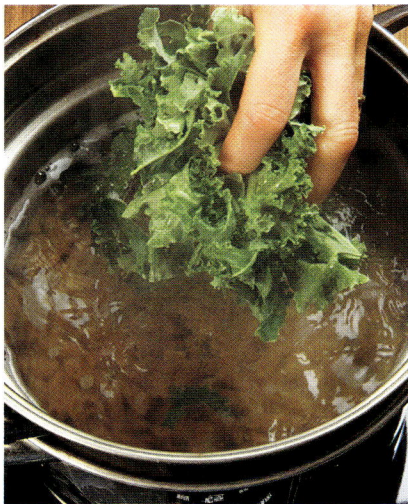

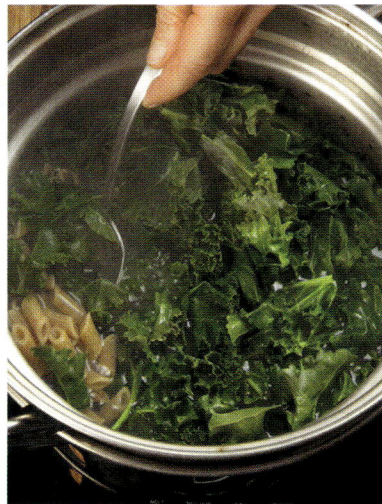

While the pasta and kale are cooking, put the pasta sauce in a pan, turn the heat to medium, cover, and heat until beginning to bubble. Reduce heat to low and keep warm until ready to use.

In a nonstick pan over medium heat, cook the zucchini until just brown. Push the zucchini aside in the pan, add the mushrooms, and continue cooking them until they soften. Remove the pan from the heat. Add drops of liquid *only* if the mushrooms and zucchini are burning.

When pasta and greens are cooked, drain and put in a large casserole dish, add hot pasta sauce, and stir. Plenty of pasta sauce is good, so extra sauce is great to have on hand.

Place the mushrooms and zucchini on top of it all and serve. Do not mix the zucchini and mushrooms into the pasta—let their flavors dance on top!

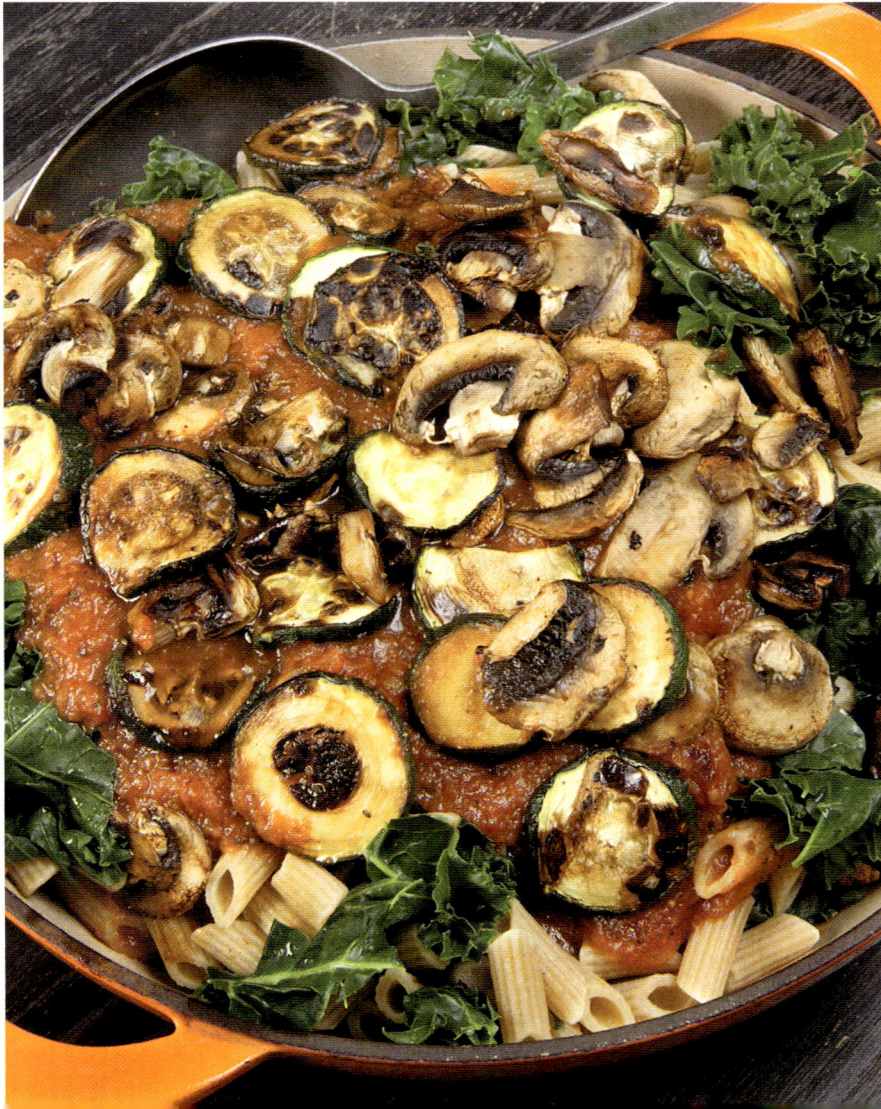

MAGNIFICENT MUSHROOM RAGOUT

A friend and wonderful cook invited us for dinner and used this recipe from Mediterranean Light *as part of a feast. Of course, we have modified it. Try dry Marsala (or port) for better flavor than red wine. If wild mushrooms are not available, use 1 pound of fresh, but be sure to use the dried for the wonderful flavor they add.*

INGREDIENTS:

1 ounce dried wild mushrooms, such as porcini or chanterelles

1 cup boiling water to cover mushrooms (reserved to use later)

1 large onion, sliced

8 ounces fresh wild mushrooms such as porcini or chanterelles (or if not available, use shiitake)

8 ounces cultivated mushrooms such as white or baby bellos, thickly sliced

4 cloves garlic, chopped

½ cup white wine or Marsala

1 cup soaking water from the dried mushrooms

½ teaspoon dried thyme

½ teaspoon dried rosemary

1 cup vegetable broth

½ teaspoon pepper

1 to 2 tablespoons low-sodium tamari, to taste (optional)

3 to 4 cups brown rice, cooked

INSTRUCTIONS:

Bring 2 cups of water to a boil.

Place dried mushrooms in a bowl. Pour boiling water over them—just enough to cover the mushrooms. Let the mushrooms soak for 30 minutes.

In a large frying pan over medium heat, cook the onions, stirring often until they are translucent and slightly browned. If the pan gets dry, add drops of wine or water if necessary. Add the fresh wild and the cultivated mushrooms; stir and cook for 5 to 10 minutes until they begin to release their liquid and brown.

Drain the dried mushrooms, but save the water—there should be about 1 cup. Shake the mushrooms a little in the colander to remove most of the water.

Add the rehydrated mushrooms to the pan along with the garlic and cook a few more minutes.

Add the wine or Marsala and bring it to a simmer.

Add the reserved soaking liquid from the mushrooms, the thyme, rosemary, and vegetable broth, and turn the heat down to a simmer again. Cover the dish and let simmer for 20 minutes. If you choose, you can eat it at this stage, or if you want a more intense flavor, uncover the mixture and raise the heat to reduce the liquid a bit.

Add pepper to taste and, if necessary, low-sodium tamari. We love this over brown rice on a bed of greens and sprinkled with parsley, but we also like it on toast, where the taste of the mushrooms is so intense. And don't forget a huge salad or Cooked Kale (page 23), as well!

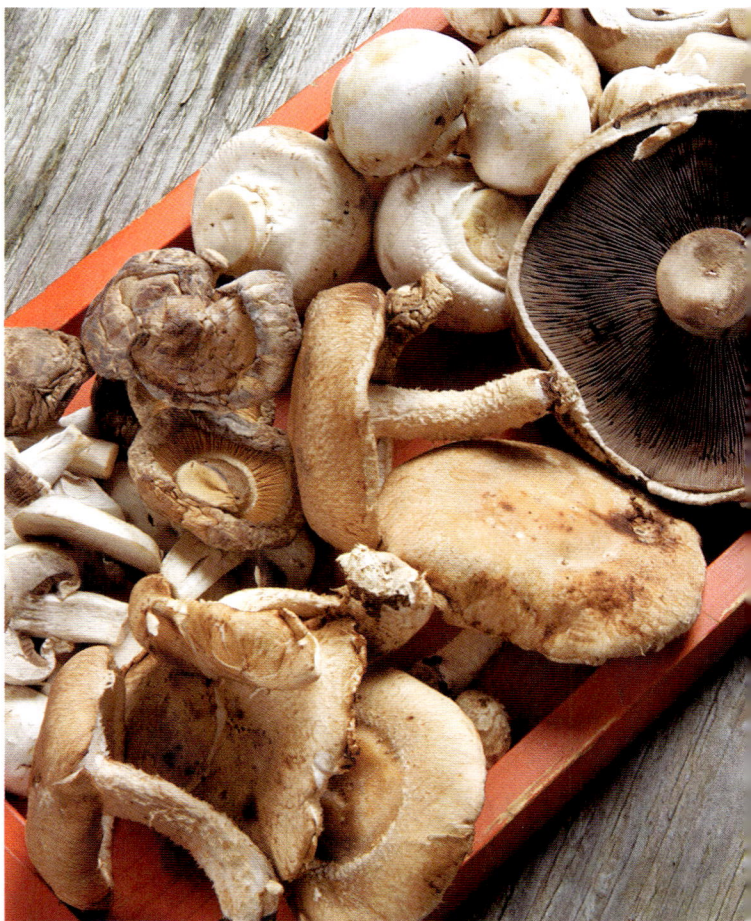

HOT (SWEET) POTATO!

This sounds crazy, but it is simple and delicious. And best of all, it's easy.

INGREDIENTS:

2 sweet potatoes, baked

1 (15-ounce) can no-salt-added black beans, drained and rinsed under hot water

1 mango, cubed

½ red bell pepper, chopped

¼ cup cilantro, chopped

3 green onions, chopped

Lime juice

INSTRUCTIONS:

Place the freshly cooked sweet potato on a plate. Cut it in half, spoon the warmed black beans onto the potato, and top with mango, red pepper, cilantro, and green onions. Squeeze lime juice over the mixture. For a larger presentation, remove potato flesh into a bowl and top with all of the ingredients. Beautiful!

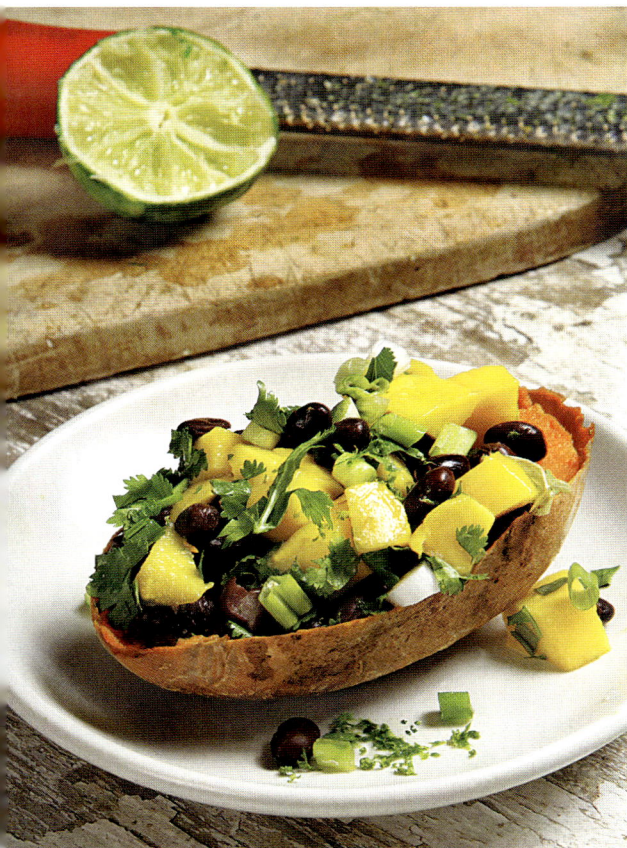

PICADILLY BOWL

Picadilly Circus is a busy meeting place in the heart of London, just as this bowl is a busy meeting place of all our favorite vegetables with the surprise addition of oats! Yes, oats and kale! You will never guess you are eating oats for dinner in this dish. Every time we have it, Essy has no idea he is eating oats for the second time in a day! Remember, oats are dose responsive, so the more you eat, the better. With asparagus and a salad, this is a fabulous and easy meal.

INGREDIENTS:

1 cup steel-cut oats

1 medium onion, chopped

4 cloves garlic, chopped

8 ounces mushrooms, sliced

1 bunch kale, stripped and chopped
  (about 4 cups)

2 cups broccoli, chopped

1 large red bell pepper, chopped

3 cups vegetable broth (we recommend
  Kitchen Basics unsalted)

6 tablespoons nutritional yeast

2 cup frozen corn (optional)

Freshly ground black pepper, to taste

8 shakes Cholula hot sauce, or to taste

INSTRUCTIONS:

In a large frying pan over medium-high heat, toast the oats until golden and fragrant, about 3 minutes. Stir frequently. Transfer to a bowl and set aside.

In the same pan over medium-high heat, add the onions and continue stirring for about 5 minutes until they soften and begin to brown. Add drops of water or vegetable broth if the pan gets too dry.

Stir in the garlic and mushrooms, and cook for 1 to 2 minutes. Again, add drops of liquid to the pan if necessary.

Rinse the kale and add to the pan while continuing to stir. Add the broccoli and bell peppers, and cook until the kale is reduced by half, about 5 minutes more.

Add the oats, broth, and nutritional yeast. Bring to a boil, cover, lower heat, and simmer for 25 minutes until most of the liquid is absorbed.

Add the corn, pepper, and Cholula hot sauce, and stir. Transfer to a casserole dish or just serve from the pan.

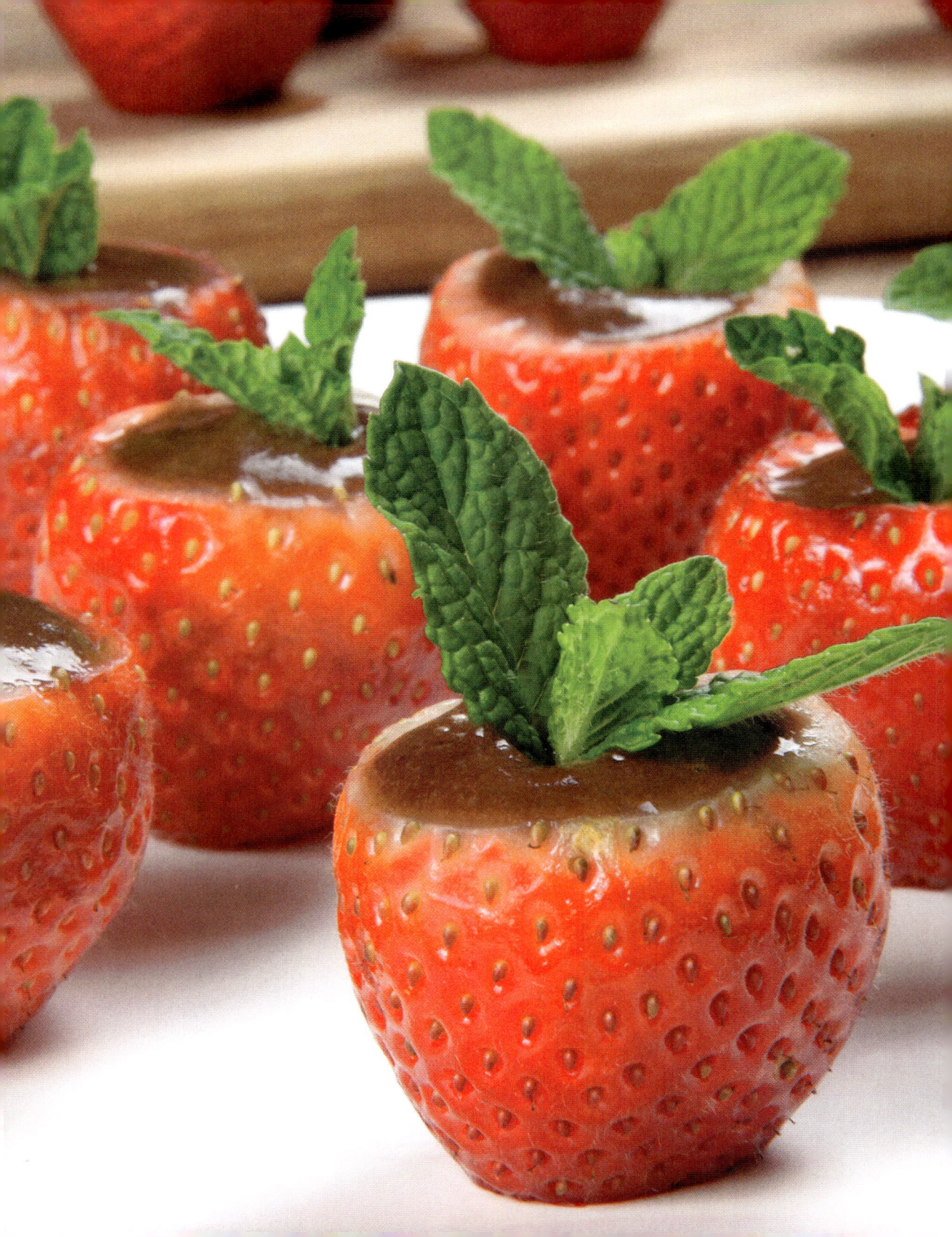

DESSERTS

Everyone loves desserts. And for some people, knowing that they can still eat dessert makes them able to embrace eating plant-based.

But, it's still best to make dessert an occasional treat and not an every night event.

Sugar is so addicting, it is hard for anyone to eat just a little. Happily, if you stop sugar for a week, you lose the craving for it. It comes back with a vengeance, however, when you take that first bite of a cookie or cake. And if you are like us, it is hard to have just one small piece.

Our desserts are sweetened only with fruit or pure maple syrup. This makes them still taste like a treat, but reasonable—not heavy, rich, or intensely sweet; just right.

We all have birthdays and special events that we love to celebrate. It's great to have a crowd over when it comes to dessert so you can divide a sweet treat into tiny pieces. We have found with many of the mousses we can make them go much further by filling them with lots of fruit so something that serves four might stretch to serve six by adding layers of bananas or berries.

Better than anything is a snack of frozen grapes. Each bite is a sweet, juicy, flavor-packed treat. Another healthy, amazing dessert is the frozen Banana Soft Serve (page 264).

FRUIT MÉLANGE

This dessert takes fruit to a sophisticated level. It is stunningly colorful and so tasty. Use a melon baller, if possible, to make the melon into balls. Melon always tastes better in little balls. Don't feel limited by the fruit we list—try others, too.

INGREDIENTS:

2 cups cantaloupe and/or honeydew, cut into ½-inch × ½-inch cubes

½ cup strawberries, sliced in half

1 cup blueberries or raspberries

1 orange, peeled and sectioned

1 kiwi, peeled and sliced

½ to 1 cup orange juice

½ teaspoon ginger, grated

½ lime, zest and juice, or to taste

6 leaves fresh mint, chiffonade

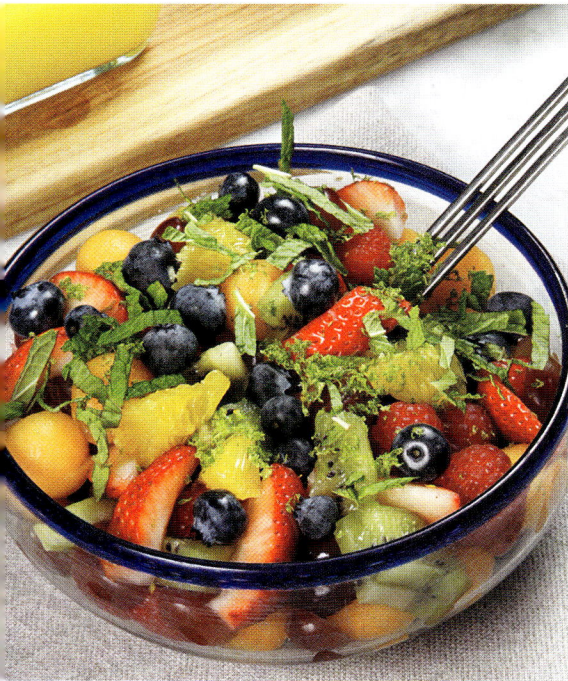

INSTRUCTIONS:

In a pretty bowl, combine melon, strawberries, blueberries, orange sections, and kiwi.

Add enough orange juice to almost cover the fruit.

Scatter the ginger and lime zest over the fruit, squeeze in the lime juice, and stir in the mint leaves.

TIP:

Try a few dollops of Raspberry Sauce (page 113) on top as a delicious addition just before serving.

4TH OF JULY FRUIT FIREWORKS

Serve this in a white bowl and it is 4th of July! This is colorful, fresh, and delicious—perfect for a summer day. Mix equal amounts of watermelon and blueberries and use plenty of fresh mint to your taste. Use a melon baller to make perfect watermelon balls. A dab of Banana Soft Serve (page 264) is the grand finale.

INGREDIENTS:

2 cups watermelon balls

2 cups blueberries

1 to 2 tablespoons fresh mint, chiffonade

INSTRUCTIONS:

Mix the watermelon, blueberries, and mint in a beautiful white bowl and serve.

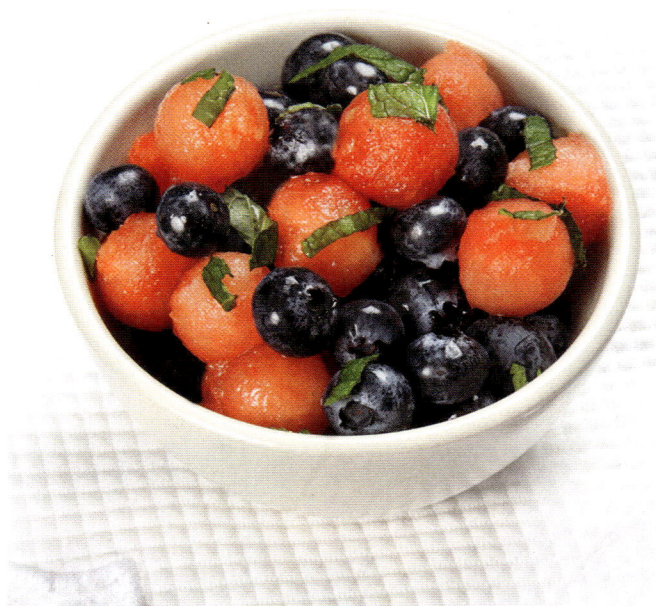

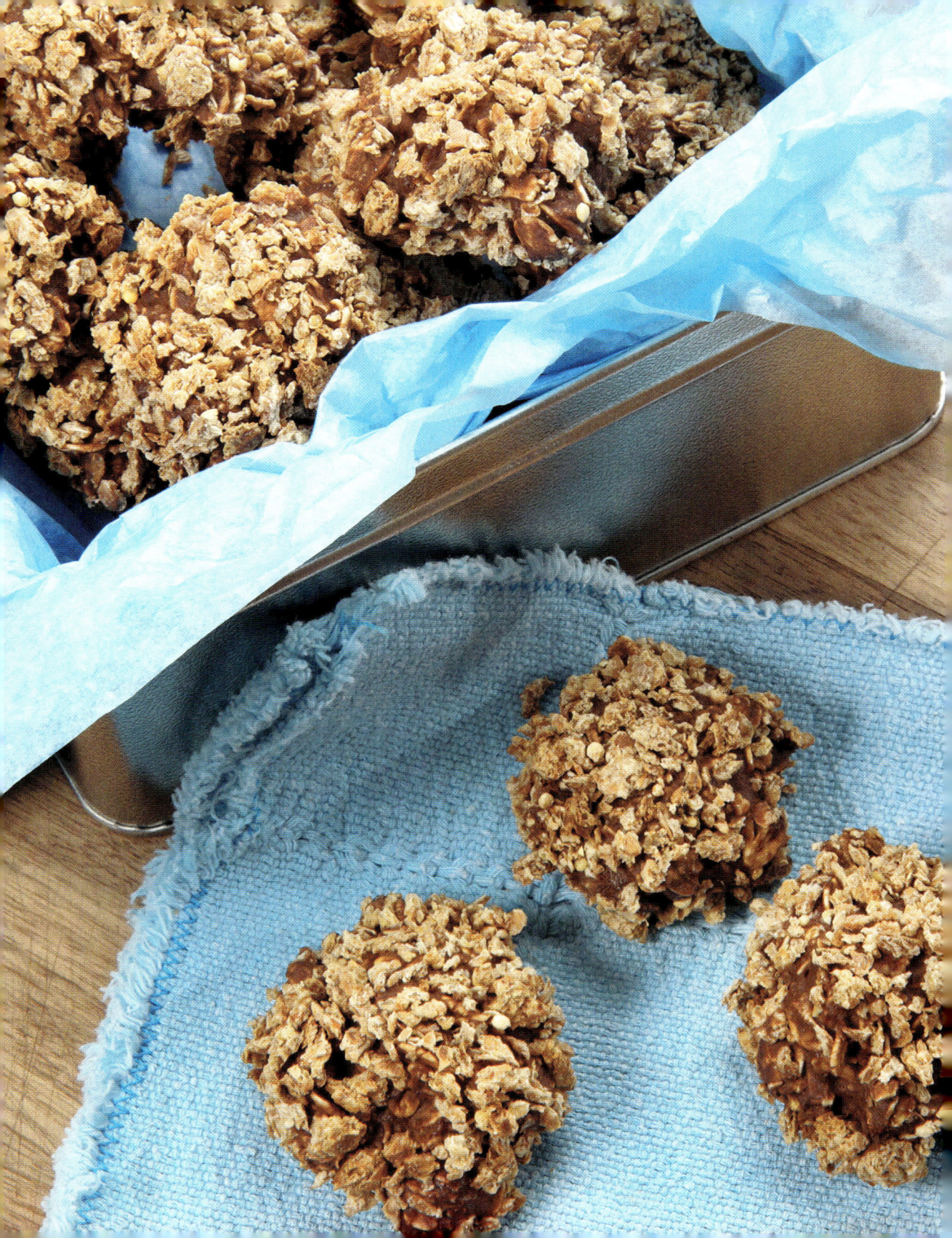

MINTY FROZEN CHOCOLATE BALLS

MAKES AROUND 40, DEPENDING ON HOW MANY YOU EAT AS YOU GO!

We think these are the healthiest, most decadent-tasting dessert treats we have had in a long time. Rolling the balls in Kashi 7 Whole Grain Nuggets helps keep the chocolate from melting on your fingers. Kashi 7 Whole Grain Nuggets are especially crunchy, but any Grape-Nuts... type nugget cereal, such as Ezekiel 4.9, works. These are delicious even if you don't roll them in a nugget cereal. They will just be sticky! No matter how you decide to make them, be sure to serve them frozen or else you'll have really, really messy fingers. They seem totally indulgent, but even if you eat them all by yourself, it's really just a lot of bananas and oats—not so awful!

INGREDIENTS:

⅓ cup cocoa powder

⅓ cup unsweetened almond milk

⅓ cup pure maple syrup, to taste

2 teaspoons pure vanilla extract

2 ripe bananas

¼ teaspoon peppermint extract

1 tablespoon chocolate balsamic vinegar or Mandarin Chocolate balsamic vinegar

2 cups oats

1 cup Kashi 7 Whole Grain Nuggets or any Grape-Nuts-like cereal

INSTRUCTIONS:

Blend all but the oats and cereal together in a food processor. Transfer to a bowl.

Add oats, and mix well.

Line a baking sheet with parchment paper or wax paper.

Put Kashi Nuggets in a small saucer with sides or a small bowl.

Using the big end of a melon baller or a small spoon, scoop up little wet, sticky chocolate balls, about the size of a large marble, one by one. Drop them in the Kashi, and with a spoon or with your fingers, gently cover the surface of the ball with nuggets. Carefully place them on the parchment paper (you may find it easiest to use your fingers). Flatten the balls slightly with the back of a spoon. Freeze. Remember to serve frozen or when they are just beginning to thaw.

MANGO MAGIC WITH RASPBERRY SAUCE

We were stunned at how easy, fast, and delicious this very simple and beautiful dessert is when our friend from Mexico, Norma, whipped it up at the very last minute just before we sat down for dinner one night. One of our granddaughters especially loves this dessert—and I make a special serving for her when we have guests.

INGREDIENTS:

2 ripe mangoes

¼ cup oat milk

4 ounces frozen unsweetened raspberries, thawed

INSTRUCTIONS:

Cut the mangoes in half, scoop out the flesh, and place into a food processor. Add the oat milk, blend, and pour into 4 individual dishes.

Place the raspberries into the blender and pulse until a smooth sauce forms.

Using a spoon, artistically spread 1 tablespoon of raspberry sauce on top of each mango bowl. We like to make the shape of the letter of the guest of honor's first name!

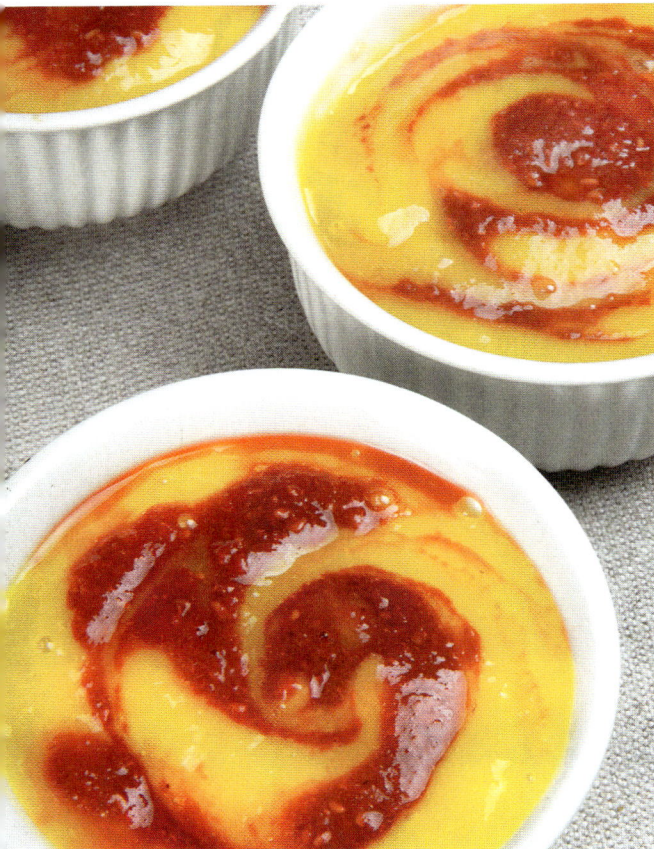

CHOCOLATE-FILLED AND LIME-KISSED STRAWBERRIES

These are fun to make, absolutely beautiful to look at, and incredibly delicious. It would be hard to make too many! Probably the clever thing to do is limit *how many each person gets. Best of all, these are only banana-sweetened; no other sweetener is used. The riper the banana, the sweeter the chocolate puree—so save those ripe old leopard-spotted wonders!*

INGREDIENTS:

12 large strawberries

1 very ripe banana

1 tablespoon unsweetened cocoa

2 teaspoons chocolate balsamic vinegar (optional)

Lime zest or mint leaves, for garnish

INSTRUCTIONS:

Slice the top off the strawberry, and then slice the tip off the bottom so the strawberry can stand on its own.

With a sharp paring knife, preferably serrated, carefully cut out the white core.

In a small food processor (if possible), puree the banana, cocoa, and chocolate balsamic vinegar, if using. Be sure to scrape down the sides so the puree is very smooth. With a small spoon, fill each strawberry with the chocolate puree.

Sprinkle lime zest or the mint leaves on the top of each strawberry.

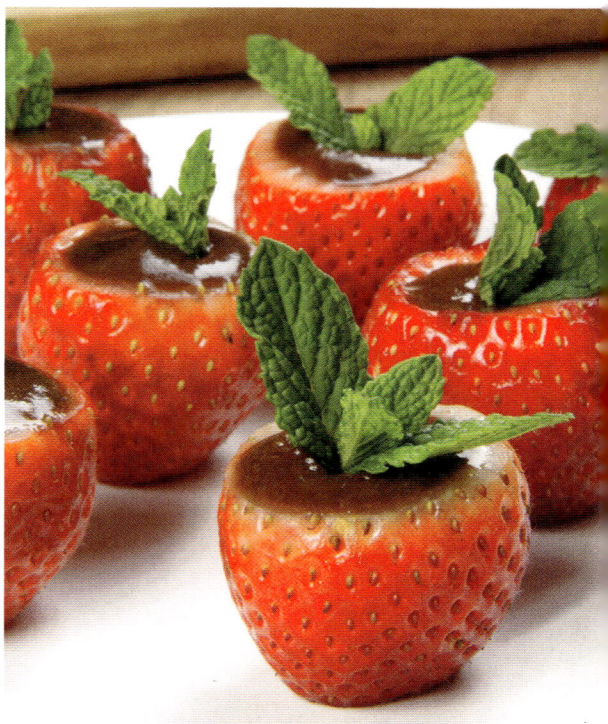

CHOCOLATE RASPBERRY-MANGO PARFAIT   SERVES 4 TO 5

We were in Bartlesville, Oklahoma, for a talk and had dinner with friends. Nancy had waited to make dessert at the last minute, and I volunteered to help since she had planned to make my chocolate mousse. I made it from memory and put in too much cocoa. Below is the result of our joint effort to resurrect it. Everyone thought it was a hit! Now it is one of our go-to desserts for guests.

INGREDIENTS:

12 ounces lite silken firm tofu

⅓ cup (or less) pure maple syrup

2 tablespoons cocoa powder

1 teaspoon pure vanilla extract

1 tablespoon chocolate balsamic vinegar

1 banana, diced

½ mango, diced, ½ cup raspberries, or both

1 cup frozen raspberries, thawed and pureed

Mint leaves, for garnish

INSTRUCTIONS:

In a food processor, blend the tofu until smooth, scraping down the sides to be sure all the tofu is well blended.

Add the maple syrup, cocoa powder, vanilla, and chocolate balsamic vinegar, and blend again.

Place the bananas in the bottom of 4 or 5 individual wineglasses or bowls, add 1 tablespoon raspberry sauce, tofu mixture, mangoes or berries, and a final tablespoon of raspberry sauce. Top with mint leaves.

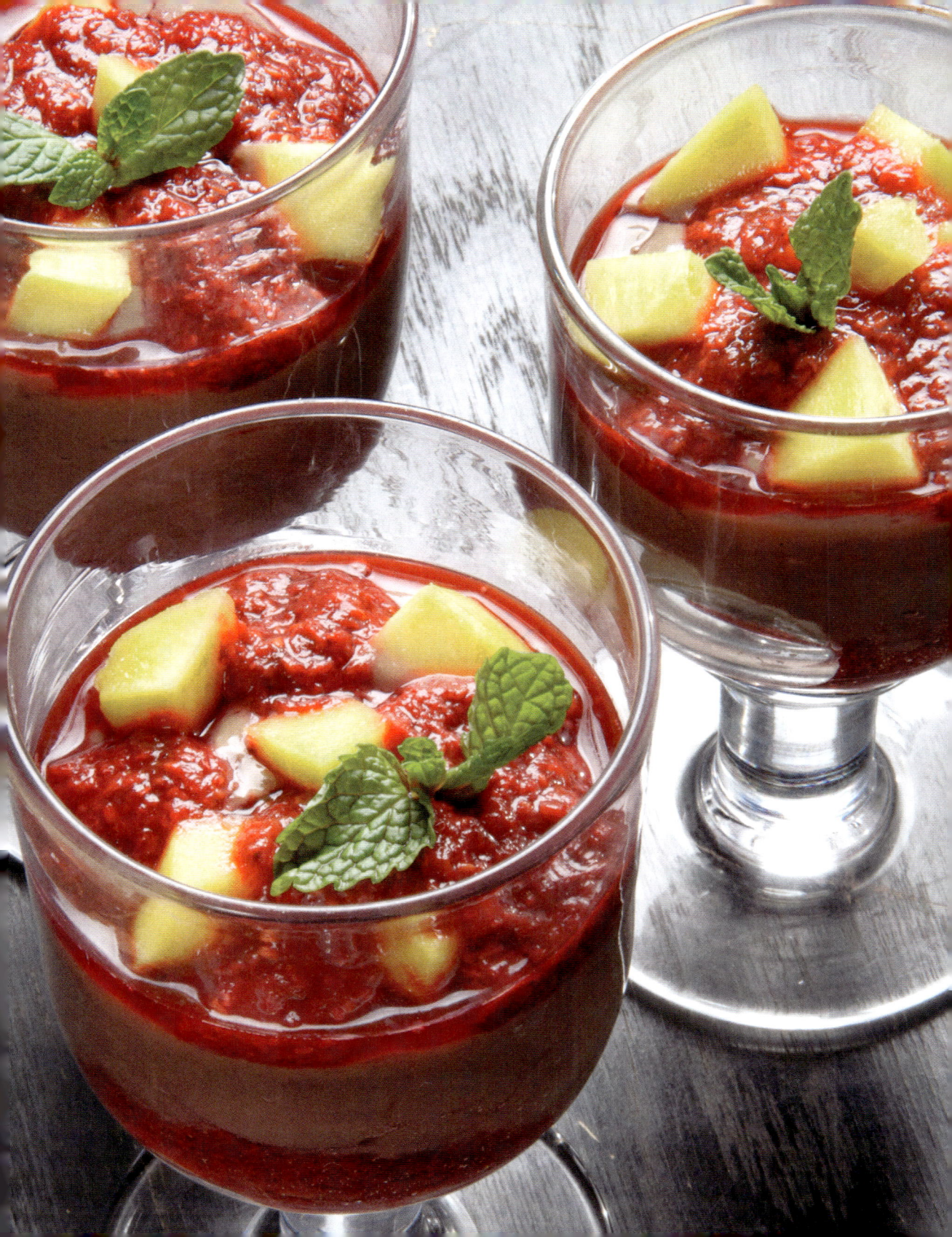

LEMON CUPCAKES WITH LIME FROSTING

I have a love affair with lemon, so when Jane arrived at our house with these moist little lemon cupcakes she had created, I was on cloud nine! They hit my lemon spot on the head! They don't rise high, so just frost them with our fantastic Lime Frosting on the following page and enjoy this bit of sunshine.

INGREDIENTS:

1½ cups oat flour (this is sometimes called oat bran flour, as well)

1 teaspoon baking soda

1 teaspoon baking powder (Hain Featherweight sodium-free, recommended)

½ cup pure maple syrup

Zest of 3 large lemons

⅔ cup fresh lemon juice

½ cup unsweetened applesauce (4 ounces)

1 teaspoon vanilla

¼ cup water

INSTRUCTIONS:

Preheat the oven to 350°F.

Line a 12-cupcake tin with paper liners or use a nonstick pan.

Combine dry ingredients in a large mixing bowl. Add the maple syrup, lemon zest and lemon juice, applesauce, vanilla, and water. Stir.

Divide batter evenly between cupcake wells. Bake for 25 to 30 minutes, until the cupcakes brown slightly. Cool, frost with Lime Frosting, and garnish with lemon zest or lime zest for a twist! They are also good unfrosted. It's that lemon punch!

LIME FROSTING

Shazam! This is alive. It works as a bright-tasting layer on Lemon Cupcakes (page 254), on Kale Cake (page 256), or alone (shh!).

INGREDIENTS:

12 ounces lite silken firm tofu

¼ cup fresh lime juice

Zest of 1 lime

⅓ cup pure maple syrup

1 tablespoon chia seeds

INSTRUCTIONS:

In a food processor combine tofu, lime juice and lime zest, and maple syrup, and blend until smooth. Be sure to scrape down the sides of the machine so all the tofu gets well blended. Add the chia seeds and pulse until the frosting is uniformly mixed. Boom, it is ready to go!

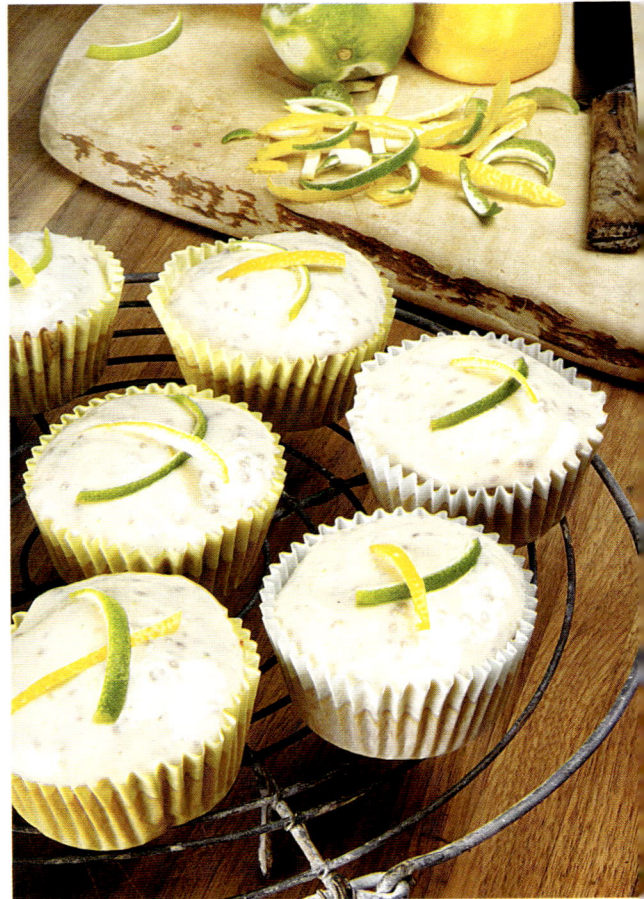

KALE CAKE WITH BLUEBERRY FROSTING

MAKES TWO 9-INCH ROUND LAYERS

That's right. Yes, we did. A kale cake! And it is great. The best response we have heard was a big "WOW" from a carnivore! Our editor prefers this with raspberry frosting. Give it a go with Lime Frosting (page 255); we love it with Blueberry Frosting (page 257). Serve with Banana Soft Serve (page 264) for that final wow.

INGREDIENTS:

4 cups raw kale, stripped, chopped, and cooked (after cooking, yields 2 cups kale)

1 cup pure maple syrup

2 teaspoons vanilla extract

½ cup unsweetened applesauce

2 tablespoons apple cider vinegar

¾ cup water

3 cups white whole wheat flour (we prefer King Arthur Flour brand)

2 teaspoons baking soda

INSTRUCTIONS:

Preheat oven to 350°F. Line two cake pans with parchment paper.

Cook the kale in a pot with 1 to 2 inches of water until the kale is dark green and soft.

Drain the kale and add it to a food processor along with the maple syrup, vanilla, applesauce, vinegar, and water.

Blend until uniformly mixed—it will look like a green smoothie at this stage.

Transfer the green goodness to a large bowl.

Add the flour and baking soda, and stir.

Pour the batter into the prepared cake pans and bake for 30 minutes. Remove the cakes from the oven and let them cool. Frost the cakes with Blueberry Frosting (page 257) or Lime Frosting (page 255), then sprinkle with blueberries and serve!

BLUEBERRY FROSTING

This powerful, purple, beautiful frosting speaks for itself. This also makes a delicious pudding sprinkled with fresh blueberries.

INGREDIENTS:

- 1 cup blueberries, fresh or frozen, or 1 cup raspberries
- ¼ cup orange juice
- 24 ounces (2 packages) lite silken firm tofu (It has to be silken and firm or you will have a runny mess or something the texture of cat litter!)
- ½ cup pure maple syrup
- 2 tablespoons chia seeds (optional)
- ½ cup fresh berries of your choice (for garnish)

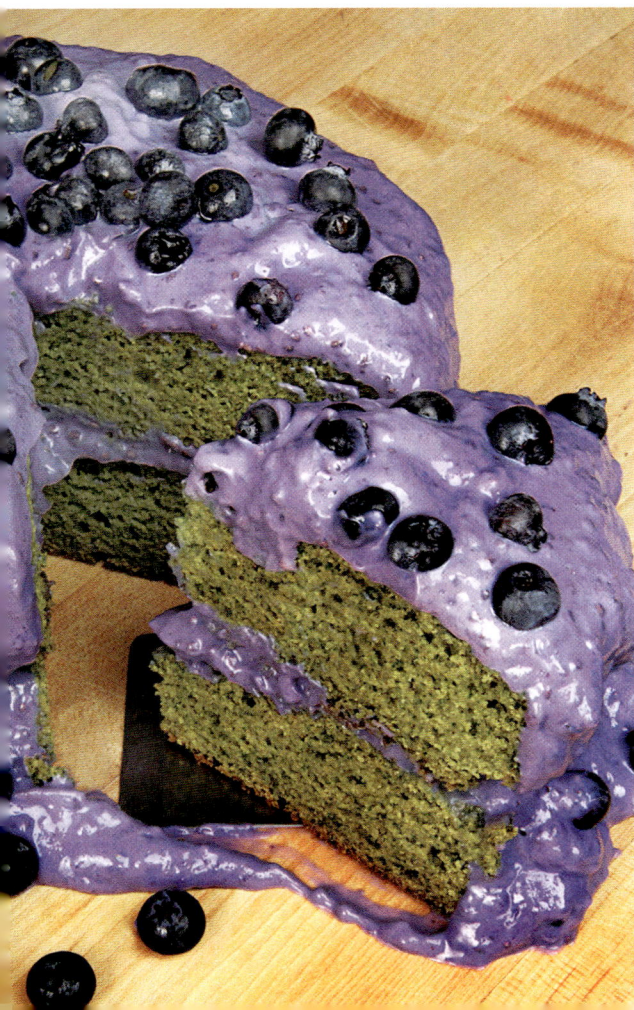

INSTRUCTIONS:

In a saucepan over high heat, boil your choice of berries and orange juice for 5 minutes. The sauce will become more syrup-like as it cooks.

Remove the sauce from the heat and pour into a food processor. Blend it until it is smooth yet with tiny bits of fruit still visible. Add the tofu, maple syrup, and chia seeds, and continue to blend until smooth.

Spread the frosting over a cake or cupcakes, or enjoy as a pudding! Garnish with fresh berries.

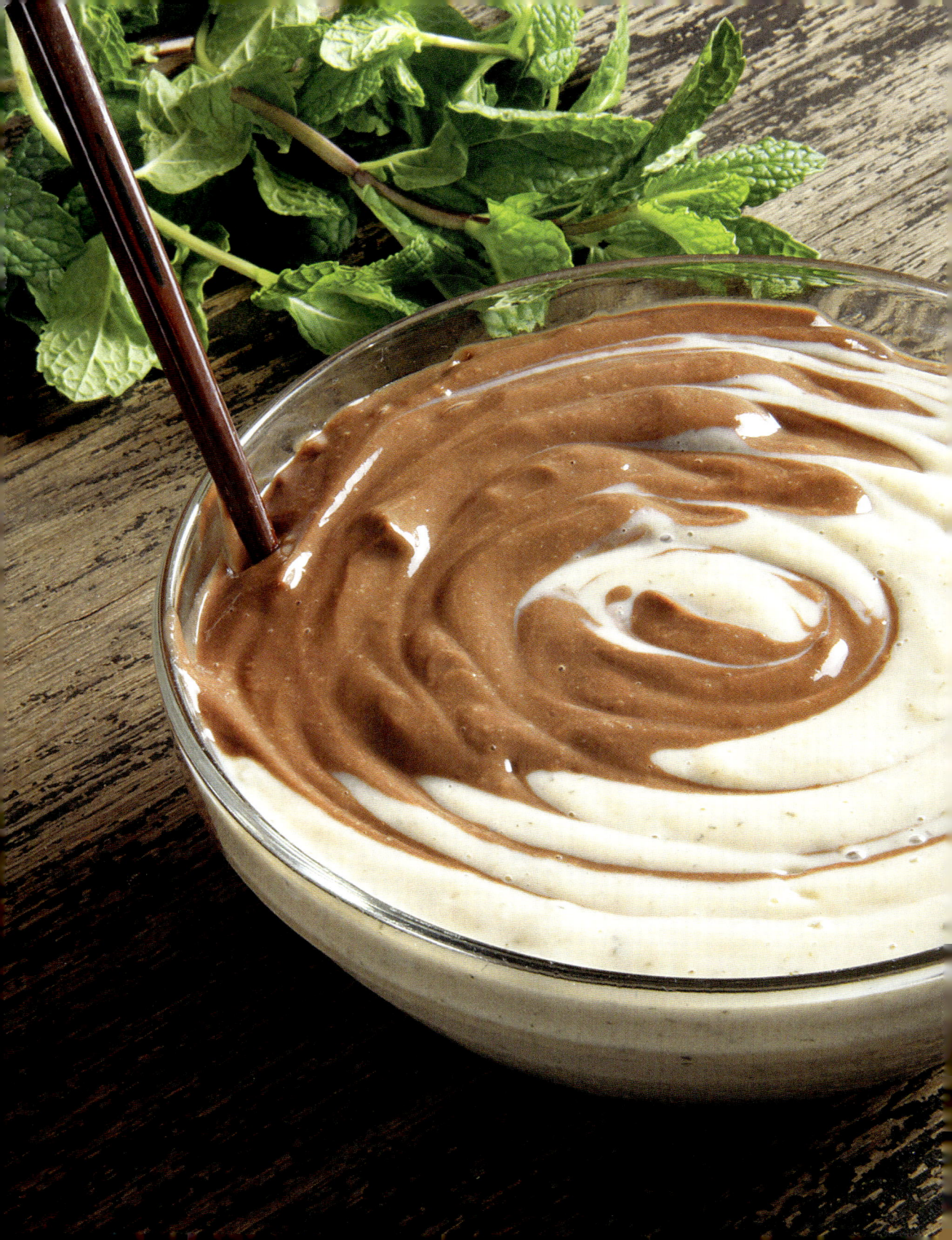

CHOCOLATE-MINT SWIRLED PUDDING

Make these two luscious recipes and swirl them together. Chocolate and mint, a match made in heaven.

CHOCOLATE INGREDIENTS:

- 12 ounces lite silken firm tofu (it has to be silken or it will come out like cat litter)
- 3 tablespoons cocoa powder
- ⅓ cup pure maple syrup
- 1 tablespoon pure vanilla extract

MINT INGREDIENTS:

- 12 ounces lite silken firm tofu
- 1 tablespoon mint leaves, minced (about 8 to 12 leaves, plus a few for garnish)
- ⅓ cup pure maple syrup
- 1 tablespoon pure vanilla extract

INSTRUCTIONS:

For the chocolate pudding: In a food processor, combine the tofu, cocoa powder, maple syrup, and vanilla, and blend until smooth. Set pudding aside and clean the food processor.

For the mint pudding: In the newly cleaned food processor, combine the tofu, mint leaves, maple syrup, and vanilla, and blend until smooth.

Into a large serving bowl, carefully pour the chocolate pudding on one side. Carefully pour the mint pudding in the other side. With a spoon, start on the chocolate pudding side and gracefully move into the mint pudding territory while shaping the letter *S*. (Or use whatever technique you prefer to lightly blend the two sides.) This will create a marbling effect between the two flavors. Chill; serve with mint leaves as garnish.

LIME CUSTARD TART WITH FRESH FRUIT

SERVES 6 TO 8

This is easy to make, heaven to eat, and looks stunning. *Use any fruit you want. It is best to assemble this shortly before eating so the crust stays crisp. It is worth searching for Kashi 7 Whole Grain Nuggets (available at health food stores) because they make such a crispy crust.*

INGREDIENTS FOR TART CRUST:

1¼ cups Kashi 7 Whole Grain Nuggets, Ezekiel 4:9, or Grape-Nuts Cereal

3 tablespoons apple or orange juice concentrate

INGREDIENTS FOR FILLING:

2 (12-ounce) packages lite silken firm or extra-firm tofu (we prefer Mori-Nu brand)

⅔ cup pure maple syrup

Zest and juice of 1 lime

6 tablespoons lime juice

1 banana, sliced

1 mango, sliced

1 cup blueberries or raspberries or both

2 kiwis, sliced

6 to 8 strawberries, sliced

INSTRUCTIONS:

Preheat the oven to 350°F.

Make the tart crust: Place the cereal and apple juice concentrate in a small bowl and stir with a fork until nuggets are moist. In a pie plate, spread the nuggets thinly over the bottom and up the sides.

Bake crust for 14 minutes, or until brown. Check often to be sure it doesn't burn.

Remove crust from oven; place in the freezer, if possible, or refrigerator until ready to fill.

Make the filling: Drain the tofu, cover with paper towels, and squeeze out any extra liquid into the towels. Place the tofu in a food processor. (Skip the squeezing if you are in a hurry and just drain. Removing some of the liquid makes the filling a little thicker.)

Place the tofu, maple syrup, lime zest, and lime juice in a mixer, and blend until very smooth. Scrape down the sides of the processor and blend completely to avoid any lumps. Refrigerate the blended tofu until ready to use.

Shortly before you are ready to serve, remove the crust from the freezer and arrange a layer of sliced bananas in the base of the crust.

Fill the crust with half the tofu mixture. Cover the tofu with 1 cup or more of mango, berries, kiwi, or fruit of choice, and then add the rest of the tofu on top of the fruit.

Finally, beautifully arrange a few slices of kiwi, strawberries, or fruit of your choice on top. The more fruit the better; you can't have too much! Be as artistic as you wish or just dump all the fruit in colorful piles.

It is especially difficult to get the first piece out of the dish. Don't even worry if none of it comes out smoothly. This tastes better in little messy heaps.

Design by Crile Hart

GINGERBREAD BISCOTTI

This yummy recipe was inspired by a JoyofBaking.com recipe with the same title—though we made some plant-based tweaks, of course. We have a variety of biscotti recipes we love, such as pumpkin biscotti and chocolate biscotti, and sometimes we add dried fruit or poppy seeds. This gingerbread recipe was our photographer's favorite!

INGREDIENTS:

1 cup old-fashioned oats, divided

1¾ cups white whole wheat flour

1 teaspoon baking powder (Hain Featherweight sodium-free recommended)

½ teaspoon baking soda

1 teaspoon ground cinnamon

½ teaspoon ground ginger

⅛ teaspoon ground cloves

½ cup pure maple syrup

¼ cup unsulfured molasses

½ teaspoon pure vanilla extract

2 tablespoons golden raisins

INSTRUCTIONS:

Preheat oven to 350°F.

Line a baking sheet with parchment paper.

In a food processor, blend ½ cup of the rolled oats until finely ground.

In a bowl, combine the finely ground oats, remaining ½ cup oats, flour, baking powder, baking soda, cinnamon, ginger, and cloves.

In a separate bowl, whisk together the maple syrup, molasses, and vanilla. Slowly add the wet mixture to the dry ingredients, and stir until combined. Scrape down the sides of the bowl as needed. Mix in the raisins until just incorporated.

Transfer the dough to a lightly floured surface and form it into a log, about 12 inches long and 3 to 4 inches wide.

Transfer the log to the prepared baking sheet, and bake for about 30 minutes or until golden brown and firm to the touch. Remove the log from the oven and let cool on a wire rack for 10 minutes.

Reduce oven temperature to 300°F. Transfer the log to a cutting board and cut it into ½- to ¾-inch-thick slices. Place the biscotti flat on the baking sheet.

Bake for 6 to 8 minutes, turn slices over, and bake for another 6 to 8 minutes or until dry and firm. Remove the biscotti from the oven and let cool, if you can stand it; it gets a bit crispier as it cools!

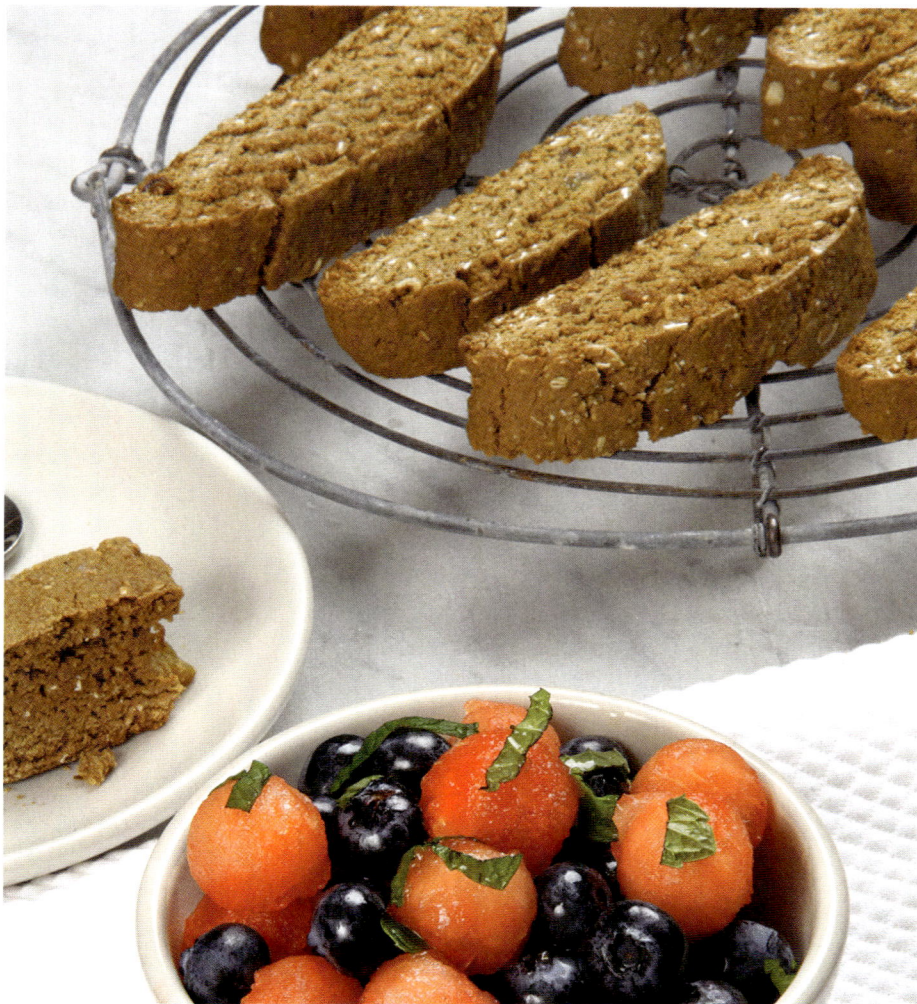

BANANA SOFT SERVE

This is so delicious—no other dessert is necessary. Have a bowl alongside your slice of Kale Cake (page 256) or anything else! You do need a strong blender or food processor; easiest of all, you can make this in a Yonanas machine or Dessert Bullet. You will never believe the magic metamorphosis from banana to creamy ice cream. Seriously, we are stunned each time we use the Yonanas machine. It is a worthwhile purchase!

If you are using a Yonanas machine, you can use whole, frozen bananas. You may need to slice the bananas into sections before you freeze them if using a different machine; check your machine's instructions.

INGREDIENTS:

1 frozen ripe banana per person (the riper the banana, the sweeter the "soft serve")

INSTRUCTIONS:

Place the bananas in the Yonanas machine (or whatever machine you are using) and be amazed at what you have created.

To eat, sprinkle with chocolate balsamic vinegar, a little pure vanilla extract, nutmeg, a sprinkle of Grape-Nuts for crunch, or all of them or none of them.

ACKNOWLEDGMENTS

We are forever grateful for the day our editors, Megan Newman and Lucia Watson, came to the farm for lunch and we plotted out this book. Very special thanks to Lucia for being our constant guiding hand and especially for her outstanding editing. And thank you, Gigi Campo, for paying attention to every little detail.

Our thanks to everyone who worked on the book, especially including our publicist, Anne Kosmoski, and publisher Brian Tart and associate publisher Lisa Johnson. And here's to the unsung heroes who helped make this book what it is: Andrea Ho, Rita Carroll, Eric Fuentecilla, Tom Consiglio, Justin Thrift, Erica Rose, Ivy McFadden, Susan Olason, Andrea Santoro, Andrea Peabbles, Gretchen Achilles, and Claire Vaccaro.

Thank you to our agent, Richard Pine, who believes in and sees things like no other!

Donna, you astounded us with your eye, your patience, and your skills—mostly the skill of seeing our food for what it is! We will now forever see food photography through the Donna Turner Ruhlman lens. In a perfect world, it would be Donna's photography alone and no need for the printed recipe.

Thanks to the inspiring Engine 2 team: Adam Riser, Jillian Gibson, Dani Little, Karen Flaherty, and Doug Lisle. You are helping to spread the word!

Our thanks to Jeff Novick for being perched on our shoulders whispering to us his extraordinary grasp of plant-based nutrition.

We could never have accomplished this book without the help of our entire family of willing supporters and tasters throughout the creation of this book. Thank you, Rip and Jill, for your ideas and always-inspiring plant-based passion. We are especially grateful to Rip for writing *The Engine 2 Diet* and *My Beef with Meat* and for the opportunity he has given us to be part of the Engine 2 team and its powerful mission. Kole, six; Sophie, four; and Hope, four weeks; have known nothing but the deliciousness of plant-based eating. Ted and Anne, you have given us ideas and been the staunchest possible supporters always. We count on you. Flinn, twenty; Gus, nineteen; and Rose, fifteen; have taken their plant-based eating with them as they move out into the world and have been wonderful ambassadors. Zeb and Polly, you have both supplied us with fabulous recipes and given us untold support. And, Georgie, eighteen months, eats the way we all wish we could eat in an ideal world where our food is prepared by loving hands other than our own. Susan Crile, sister and aunt, thank you for your ideas, artistic eye, and encouragement.

Brian, son-in-law and husband, has been our tasting guide, naysayer, and recipe saver. His food wisdom has rescued many a day. Crile, fifteen; Zeb, fourteen; and Bainon, twelve; have expanded their plant-based palates as they have tasted new dishes that seemed to appear daily on their dinner table these past recipe-creating months.

Finally, Essy! He is the reason we have had the pleasure of creating this book. He has bucked the years of criticism and stood strong in his confidence that the science shows whole-food, plant-based nutrition halts and selectively reverses heart disease. He has the patience to talk endlessly to people on the phone and most especially he cares deeply about spreading the message of the power of whole-food, plant-based nutrition. To him our *huge* thanks and enormous *love*!

INDEX

Page numbers in *italics* indicate photographs.

The *New York Times* bestseller that can both help prevent and reverse the effects of heart disease

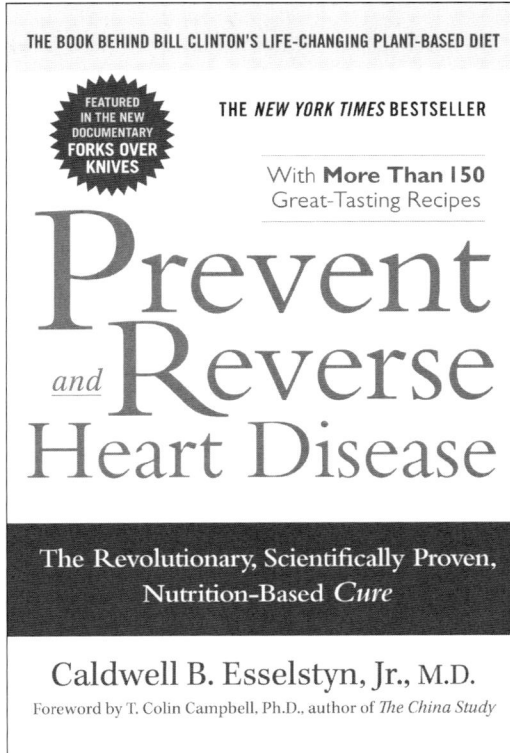

THE BOOK BEHIND BILL CLINTON'S LIFE-CHANGING PLANT-BASED DIET

FEATURED IN THE NEW DOCUMENTARY **FORKS OVER KNIVES**

THE *NEW YORK TIMES* BESTSELLER

With **More Than 150** Great-Tasting Recipes

Prevent *and* Reverse Heart Disease

The Revolutionary, Scientifically Proven, Nutrition-Based *Cure*

Caldwell B. Esselstyn, Jr., M.D.

Foreword by T. Colin Campbell, Ph.D., author of *The China Study*

Based on the groundbreaking results of his twenty-year nutritional study, *Prevent and Reverse Heart Disease* by Dr. Caldwell Esselstyn, Jr., illustrates that a plant-based, oil-free diet can not only prevent the progression of heart disease but can also reverse its effects.

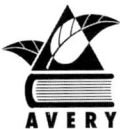

AVERY